The Doctor's Communication Handbook

I0875892

Of Previous Editions:

> "... breaks new ground in its readability ... It is concise, wise, and firmly pragmatic".
>
> *British Medical Journal*

> "Since it was first published in 1994, Peter Tate's *The Doctor's Communication Handbook* has been essential reading to improve GP registrars' communication skills".
>
> *Practical Diabetes International*

This essential text for doctors in both general practice and hospital medicine has established itself as the ultimate guide to patient communication, whatever their experience and wherever they practise. Highly respected and acclaimed for its light, conversational tone, this ninth edition, completely updated and expanded by the current authors, is revised for a broader audience to include any allied health professionals consulting with patients across the NHS and other healthcare systems.

Key Features:

- Unique and accessible approach to this vital and frequently poorly practised aspect of medicine.
- Covers all types of consultation, including telephone triage and both in-person and virtual consultation, with their associated risks and benefits.
- Explores the impact of AI, the internet, and social media on the consultation – and why doctors need not feel fazed by it.
- Addresses the change in practice where traditional doctor consultations are increasingly undertaken by other health professionals, including nurse practitioners and paramedics.
- Retains all the features praised in previous editions – brevity, readability, and humour – while being reorganised and updated by the new author team for a fresh and current approach.

The Doctor's Communication Handbook continues to provide an invaluable "one stop shop" to help students, practising doctors, nurses, and other healthcare practitioners value and improve their skills in this critical area of practice.

The Doctor's Communication Handbook

Ninth Edition

Francesca Frame

Peter Tate

Phil Whitaker

CRC Press
Taylor & Francis Group
Boca Raton London New York

CRC Press is an imprint of the
Taylor & Francis Group, an **informa** business

Designed cover image: Shutterstock

Ninth edition published 2027
by CRC Press
2385 NW Executive Center Drive, Suite 320, Boca Raton FL 33431

and by CRC Press
4 Park Square, Milton Park, Abingdon, Oxon, OX14 4RN

CRC Press is an imprint of Taylor & Francis Group, LLC

ISBN: 9781041098560 (hbk)
ISBN: 9781041109662 (pbk)
ISBN: 9781003652137 (ebk)

DOI: 10.1201/9781003652137

Typeset in Bembo
by Deanta Global Publishing Services, Chennai, India

Contents

About the authors

Francesca Frame qualified in medicine from Cambridge University in 2006 and works as a GP partner in a rural Cambridgeshire practice. In addition to her clinical work, for the past nine years she has also been an elected member of her Local Medical Committee (LMC), which works to represent, support, and advise GPs in her area. This role has brought the opportunity to attend and speak at multiple national LMC conferences, across a range of topics affecting GPs. Francesca was the co-author of the eighth edition of *The Doctor's Communication Handbook* with Peter Tate in 2019, and the co-author of *Bedside Matters*, also with Peter Tate (CRC Press, 2021).

Peter Tate qualified as a doctor at Newcastle in 1968. After spells as a P&O surgeon and as a trainee in Kentish Town, he was a family doctor in Abingdon for 30 years, a trainer for 25 of those years. From 1981 to 2006, he worked for the MRCGP exam and retired as Chief Examiner. He was awarded the MBE for services to general medical practice in 2008. The first edition of *The Doctor's Communication Handbook* was published in 1994 by Radcliffe Medical Press. He wrote *The Other Side of Medicine*, a collection of essays (Radcliffe Publishing Ltd, 2007) and *Bedside Matters*, an autobiography (CRC Press, 2021) with Francesca Frame as co-author. He was also a co-author of *The Consultation: An Approach to Learning and Teaching* (OUP, 1983) and *The New Consultation* (OUP, 2003).

Phil Whitaker qualified in medicine at Nottingham University in 1990 and has over 30 years' experience as a GP, 15 of them also acting as an educational supervisor (GP trainer). In addition to his clinical roles, he is the medical editor of the *New Statesman*, where he has been writing about medicine and health since 2013. He is the author of *What is a Doctor?* (Canongate, 2023), which uses narrative non-fiction to explore the seismic changes in the medical profession since he qualified. Alongside his medical writing, he has published six novels and won several literary awards. He was made a Fellow of the Royal College of General Practitioners in 2024.

Preface

I wrote the first edition of this book over a weekend in 1993, probably while listening to Joni Mitchell singing "you don't know what you have got 'til it's gone".

At that time I was working with a group of colleagues on the Royal College of General Practitioners' membership exam (the MRCGP), and we wanted to use the opportunity to push patient-centred medicine to the fore, reasoning that doctors took matters more seriously if they were examined. We created an examination based on direct observation of actual performance, recorded on videotape. The technology was very clunky, the exam irritated many trainers, examiners, and candidates alike, but it did change the culture a little bit, and the fact that this guide to consulting has made it to a ninth edition is something I am proud of.

Two other people I am very proud of are the current authors. Phil Whitaker was my registrar in the 1990s and is still a GP as well as a writer and influential commentator on medical issues. Francesca Frame wrote the previous edition with me and is an active GP, friend, and wise counsel.

What did I have as a GP when the first edition appeared? Almost all patient contacts were face to face, with a significant proportion held in the patient's home. I had been in practice for 20 years by 1993, and had delivered a good number of those registered with me. GPs were responsible for their own patient list 24 hours a day, and often climbed out of bed to visit sick patients.

The consultation back then was relatively unencumbered with any preventive agenda; this was several years before QOF (Quality and Outcomes Framework, the method by which GP practices are funded, based on achieving certain clinical measures and standards), and both patient and doctor (only doctors in those days) were much freer to choose and discuss their own agendas. I have to say I loved my job.

My first pacemaker was inserted in 1976, half a century ago, so I have lived that time as a patient too, which has kept me in touch with medicine at the coalface. This led me to David Pendleton along with other notable enthusiasts, and eventually to publishing *The Consultation: An Approach to Learning and Teaching*, where we championed doctors seeking out the belief systems of their patients and trying to achieve a shared understanding; a very personalised medicine, centred on the individual.

Now, only a third of a century since the first edition, the medical milieu has changed almost beyond recognition. No single event has occurred to explain such a change, and the response to COVID-19 only exaggerated and brutalised the trends which were already taking place. It is as if I had gone to sleep at the millennium dreaming of my imperfect but halcyon elysian field of primary care, and then woke up in 2026 only to find "they paved paradise, put up a parking lot".

I qualified aged 21 and am now 80, so have had plenty of time to mull over medical things. In 1986, I was lucky enough to work for a few months at the Department of Human Values in Medicine at The University of South Florida in St Petersburg, what they then called *ethics* in the States. I was teaching medical communication but, for the first time, was forced to consider the underpinning assumptions of Western medicine.

There is no easy fix to restore true patient-centred medicine, but the medical profession must consider the ethical framework that it is subscribing to. During my career, medicine was practised under a Judaeo-Christian deontological framework, with most doctors working under a time-honoured role of beneficent paternalism. Utilitarian John Stuart Mill and the like railed for the rights of the individual while being aware of the greater good, and in the latter half of the 20th century there was a distinct tilt in that direction, of which this book was a very small part. But other drivers emerged, a centrally driven, some might say totalitarian, ethic appeared, where medical agendas were imposed, no arguments were brooked, and meaningful, shared understanding in a consultation became very hard to achieve. Words like *misinformation* crept into the lexicon, the public was told that science must not be questioned, and experts were always right. There has been no real debate about this shift in UK medical circles, which is shameful. One of my favourite medical books of the 1980s about medical communication, *Meetings Between Experts*, advocated that achieving a shared understanding should be the goal of the medical encounter. Here the expert, the clinician, could be challenged, softened and even corrected by those that knew more about their beliefs, their knowledge, and their understanding.

With Covid, access to medical care became more remote, and for patients, meaningful conversations with their clinicians became harder to achieve. This little handbook gives you some of the tools to fight back, and we really do need to fight back. This book might make you stop and think about your values, and what sort of clinician you wish to be.

We must reinstate honesty as a prime driver; not as a dictat, but as an area with fuzzy edges. To re-establish trust, our patients must see us at least struggling with the issues that true, full medical disclosure raises. Plastering the cracks of uncertainty with fabricated cant helps no one. We must try to understand the people who consult with us, and to do that we have to be kind, curious, skilled, and – often difficult – involved. *Tout comprendre, c'est tout pardonner*. It may be that patients might now reverse this French expression. Should we have been braver over recent years, more the patient's advocate, less dogmatic and far less defensive?

There seems to be less kindness in the world, but clinicians caring about their patients, the lives they live, their search for happiness, and the beliefs they have are a good base. Read this book, think about yourself as a clinician, then practise the skills to improve your communication, and you will be surprised by the joy this gives you. Yes, this is a selfish aim, but the side effects of your happiness will be to make your patients more able to cope, while your diagnostic acumen will improve exponentially.

Good reading.

Peter Tate MBE
Dorchester

References

Pendleton D et al. *The Consultation: An Approach to Learning and Teaching*, Oxford University Press 1984.

Tuckett D et al. *Meetings Between Experts: An Approach to Sharing Ideas in Medical Consultations*, Tavistock Publications, 1985.

CHAPTER

1 Mattering

Clinicians, and those who train them, should learn how to ask less, "What is the matter with you?" and more, "What matters to you?"

Don Berwick, 2016

Peter Tate wrote the first edition of *The Doctor's Communication Handbook* (*DCH*) in 1994. Initially written as an examination aid for the Membership of the Royal College of General Practitioners (MRCGP) exam, this project became his love letter to the art of practising medicine, which has been his life's work and passion.

Peter's father was a GP who ran what we would now call an "old-school" general practice: a single-hander, responsible for his patients 24 hours a day, with a basement surgery and Peter's mother filling the role of receptionist, secretary, and nurse. Despite the hardship of the role, he loved his job, and observing his father's work began Peter's appreciation of the power of continuity, trust, and effective communication in the relationship between a doctor and a patient. A patient at his father's funeral told Peter that his father had been a special GP "because he always listened, he always knew what mattered". This was another era of medicine, a different world to the one we work in today, yet so much remains relevant.

Peter's appreciation of "mattering" grew during his time as a GP and GP trainer. However, as with so many of us, the real dawning of realisation came

DOI: 10.1201/9781003652137-1

during Peter's own experiences, earned during multiple admissions with cardiac arrhythmia and infective endocarditis. He experienced first-hand the army of doctors around the bed refusing to make eye contact, the bad news broken with British irony and euphemism, and a distinct lack of clear information or any attempt to seek Peter's perspective. And this was not just the experience of the awkward communication with a fellow doctor, but something Peter witnessed again and again with the patients in the beds around him. This was paternalistic, doctor-focused communication, with patients as passive recipients of whatever the doctors felt was right for them, irrespective of whether they even understood what was happening.

This personal experience of the inadequacy of typical doctor–patient communication added further impetus to Peter's growing feeling that doctors could do a much better job of understanding and responding to what really matters to their patients. A fortunate meeting with psychologist David Pendleton developed into a sabbatical at Oxford University's Department of Experimental Psychology. This academic work alongside David Pendleton, and fellow GP trainers Theo Schofield and David Havelock, led to the development of ICE – the "ideas, concerns, and expectations" mnemonic which has haunted many a clinical examinee, but which represents a powerful tool that develops an appreciation of the true essence of a consultation. The four researchers detailed their findings in their seminal 1984 book *The Consultation*. Their key message was that the true purpose of any consultation was for both parties to *achieve as genuine a shared understanding* as possible.

Peter went on to write *DCH*, originally an examination guide for GP trainees undertaking MRCGP, but which became a widely respected text on the fundamental importance of genuine communication in a truly effective consultation – why it matters and how we can learn to use its power for the benefit of our patients. It also recognised that this is a skill, something to be practised, worked at, and developed with time and experience. Here was behavioural psychology applied to medical practice. Peter identified the three main internal drivers that made up the very essence of consulting. First and perhaps most important is *curiosity* – a desire to discover what really matters to your patient. This leads, second, to a need to help your patients to *understand*, which leads, third, to the development of *trust*. Peter's work was fundamental in reshaping the teaching and practice of a generation of doctors.

The health service that Peter and his father worked in has changed dramatically. Where previous doctors, particularly GPs, had multiple opportunities to build an understanding relationship with their patients, in the modern-day health service we may have only one chance to get it right. As medicine becomes more fragmented, more pressured, and continuity is lost, effective consultations matter more than ever.

Never has the pace of change in consulting been as rapid as now. The eighth edition of *DCH* (published in 2019) explored the difference that the explosion of readily available information has brought to the consultation – doctors as the interpreters of unfiltered medical information that patients can access with just a few swipes; doctors as the explainers and contextualisers rather than the source of knowledge. In 2019, we were already grappling with increasing demand, greater medical complexity, and increasing medical workload leading to less time with our patients, when an unexpected challenge arrived. None of us had heard of SARS-CoV-2, which changed the world almost overnight, and medical practice with it. Consultations, which were previously overwhelmingly carried out face to face, switched to telephone, video, or virtual e-consults. Consulting habits and behaviours established over careers had to handbrake-turn into new patterns and new ways of working. Six years later, UK general practice and hospitals alike are creaking under the strain of demand, workload, and a burnt-out, shrinking workforce. With fewer doctors and more patients, consultations are changing again. Patients now consult with a greater variety of healthcare professionals than ever before, sometimes as well as seeing a doctor, at other times instead of. Continuity of care is becoming further fractured and fragmented, and medical practice seems to be inexorably moving from relationship medicine to transactional medicine.

With this edition we want to recognise and explore the changing landscape of the last six years and bring *DCH* in line with modern-day clinical practice. The art of good consulting is no longer the domain of just the doctor, but of anyone who consults with a patient. The content of this book remains highly pertinent, whether at the beginning of your training when establishing your skills, or as an experienced clinician. It is also relevant no matter where you work: busy emergency departments, hospital wards, or community general practice; anywhere a patient talks to a clinician. What matters is the shared understanding and goals reached by two individuals who try to understand each other from their own unique perspectives. Patients want to be listened to, and the art of effective communication alone has significant therapeutic benefits. The key messages within *DCH* are, we believe, more important now than they ever have been.

A quick word about terminology. Considering the skill mix in today's health service, we agonised about changing the title and semantics of our text, perhaps calling this new edition something like *The Clinician's Communication Handbook* to better reflect what has become a wider audience for this work. Set against this is the long history and reputation of *DCH* as a "brand", together with the fact that much of the source material we draw on focuses on clinical encounters with doctors. We ultimately decided to honour tradition with our title but have used the terms "doctor" and "clinician" interchangeably throughout the text to emphasise this book's relevance and importance to all who consult with patients. If our choice of terminology causes any offence to anyone of any professional background, we can only apologise and ask for understanding.

Peter and his father both qualified from Durham University School of Medicine in Newcastle (now part of Newcastle University) where the paediatrician Sir James Spence practised, and who said:

> *The real work of a doctor is not an affair of health centres, or laboratories, or hospital beds. Techniques have their place in medicine, but they are not medicine. The essential unit of medical practice is the occasion when, in the intimacy of the consulting room or sick room, a person who is ill, or believes himself to be ill, seeks the advice of a doctor whom he trusts. This is a consultation, and all else in the practice of medicine derives from it.*
>
> **(Spence, 1960)**

The medical world of today is different from that of Peter and his father, but when you pare it all back, the fundamentals of the consultation have not changed. There is still a clinician talking to a patient, with the sole aim of eliciting not just what illness they have, but what matters. And, as we shall discover, understanding what matters has never mattered more.

References

Berwick DM. Era 3 for Medicine and Health Care. *JAMA*. 2016;315(13):1329–1330. doi:10.1001/jama.2016.1509

Pendleton D, et al. *The Consultation: an approach to learning and teaching*. Oxford University Press; 1984.

Spence J. The need for understanding the individual as a part of the training and functions of doctors and nurses [speech delivered at a conference on mental health, March 1949]. In: *The Purpose and Practice of Medicine: Selections from the Writings of Sir James Spence*. London: Oxford University Press; 1960. p. 273–274.

CHAPTER

2

The Patient and What Matters to Them

The greatest mistake in medicine is to treat the diagnosis rather than the patient.

Eugene Braunwald

- ICE is the foundation of good communication, not a tick-box exercise.
- Understanding the patient in front of you avoids dysfunctional consultations.
- Clinicians hold power and control in the consultation, but this needs to be used effectively.
- Continuity of care matters and should be promoted and prioritised.

The mnemonic "ideas, concerns, and expectations", or ICE, was coined by Peter and his colleagues during their work in the 1980s and 1990s. Since its inception, ICE has perfectly captured the focus required for effective and efficient communication, but sadly for many it has become reduced to a tick-box exercise – at one of our local hospitals, discharge letters now baldly state "Patient's ICE – met".

One of the factors in this reduction is a perceived lack of time and capacity to fully explore ICE. For some clinicians, attending to ICE can feel like a "nice to have" rather than the key to time-efficient (and holistic) medical interactions. As the healthcare workforce expands, and many more allied healthcare

DOI: 10.1201/9781003652137-2

professionals are now consulting independently, it is worth revisiting why eliciting and exploring a patient's ICE matters for both effective and efficient consulting. First, let's focus on the factors that influence the clinician's consulting choices, and what matters to them.

Historically, medicine has been delivered in a paternalistic, doctor-centred and doctor-driven manner for centuries. Modern medical consultations will now be almost unrecognisable to those practising 50 years ago, until you look at the fundamental basis of every interaction: learning and understanding what matters to the patient in front of you. To do this, we need to understand the role of agendas, power, and control within the consultation.

Agendas

One approach to thinking about the ways in which we communicate is to consider the *agendas* for both the healthcare professional and patient. Figure 2.1

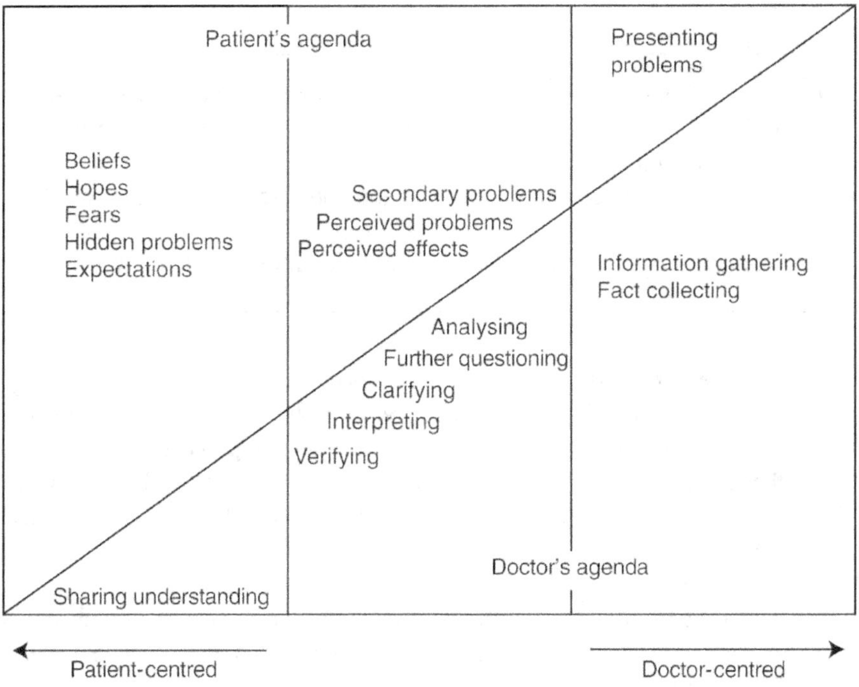

FIGURE 2.1 A power-shift model of styles of consultation.

demonstrates diagrammatically the possible spectrum of our communication behaviour with patients.

The right-hand side of the diagram is nearly all our agenda, with only the presenting complaint coming from the patient. As the communication style moves to the left, more and more of the patient's agenda is taken on board, until at the left-hand end of the diagram it is nearly all the patient's agenda. Most of us tend towards the right-hand end of this model.

The whole act of *taking* a history is a clinician-centred agenda, and this is not necessarily bad. Medical thoroughness and good pattern recognition are a hallmark of this style when practised well. As an example of clinician-centred agenda, imagine the fictitious Mrs Arthur's first GP appointment. It could go something like this:

Clinician Good morning, Mrs Arthur. I believe you are here about a neck lump. Tell me, have you lost weight?
Mrs A No.
Clinician Any hot flushes?
Mrs A No.
Clinician Feeling tired or slowed up?
Mrs A Er, well, maybe a little.
Clinician Bowels OK? Not constipated are you?
Mrs A Not really, I was wondering …

Clinician I think I should examine you now. Would you take your shirt off …?
Mrs Arthur's agenda has not figured in the conversation so far – only the clinician's agenda is being addressed.

Imagine this shift to the left of the diagram, using the same scenario:

Clinician Good morning, Mrs Arthur. I believe you are here about a neck lump. Would you tell me about it?
Mrs A Oh, er, well yes, I first noticed the swelling a few months ago, but I didn't do anything about it for a while.
Clinician Why not?
Mrs A Oh, you know, I hoped it would go away while fearing the worst.
Clinician The worst?
Mrs A Cancer, what else?
Clinician That's a frightening thought. Do you still think it may be cancer?
Mrs A Well, yes, but I'm hoping you will be able to tell me.

Here, the patient's agenda figures highly to start with, and the clinician has not yet started on their agenda.

The totally patient-centred clinician is probably a dangerous creature. Patients do, after all, come to us for medical advice and considered professional opinions. They do not generally expect us to let them do all the talking, planning, and managing (although, in rare cases, this may be appropriate). An ideal might perhaps lie around the middle of this spectrum, changing behaviour one way or the other depending on the needs of the patient and the situation. The problem, however, as shown by experience and research, is that generally we *do not change*. Recordings of multiple consultations by the same doctor (during the era of video-MRCGP exams) showed a remarkable consistency of style. Thus, we say and do things in much the same way with an anxious 16-year-old coming for contraception as with a 50-year-old woman with menorrhagia or an 80-year-old woman with vulval carcinoma. It appears that we do not regularly adapt to meet the needs of the patient; our agendas are fixed. You could say that this does not matter so long as we have an effective set of behaviours with which we can cope with most patients, but later in this chapter we will find that different patients need different types of communication. We need to be flexible, and it appears that most of us are not.

Our basic agenda is to discover why our patient has come to see us. This seems almost too obvious to state, but in many consultations clinicians and patients do not appear to be talking about the same thing. Years ago, one of the great academic GPs, Professor Pat Byrne, gave this type of communication the deliberately ugly name of *dysfunctional*. In this sort of consultation, the clinician and the patient are each pursuing their own quite separate agendas.

Dysfunctional communication is common in all areas of medical practice. Consider the case of Mrs Arthur again. Let us carry on with the clinician-centred example. Assume that the clinician has examined Mrs Arthur and completed the history taking in the form of a series of closed questions. Mrs Arthur has therefore contributed none of her own thoughts and feelings. The time for explanation and management has come.

Clinician Well, Mrs Arthur, there is nothing to worry about. You probably have a multinodular goitre, which is usually a benign condition. There are a couple more tests we need to do just to be on the safe side. I will arrange a referral for a scan and biopsy of that biggish lump. Is that OK?

Mrs A So you are sure it is not serious?

Clinician I'm sure it's not, but the hospital will be seeing you soon. Goodbye.
Mrs A Well, goodbye, er, thank you.

This is deficient communication. Consider her ICE; Mrs Arthur has not had any of her agenda addressed. She will probably attend the tests out of fear, but she may not attend at all as it seems too scary. She is not sure what the words "multinodular", "goitre", "benign", "scan", or "biopsy" mean, and she will go home feeling frustrated and afraid. The clinician, in turn, has focused their attention on the thyroid gland to the exclusion of everything else. The clinician knows little about Mrs Arthur and nothing about her specific fears or reasons for consulting. This encounter is truly dysfunctional.

Clinicians are good at diagnosis (i.e. establishing in the medical sense why a patient has come to see them). We discover the nature and history of the problem and the likely cause, but we tend not to be good at searching out our patients' beliefs and expectations. These are the real reasons why patients come to see us, and not discovering them can lead to a mismatch of agendas. Eliciting the patient's agenda is particularly challenging in time-pressured scenarios (though ironically it usually saves time in the long run), but not uncovering the patient's agenda risks not engaging them, leading to them not following medical advice and treatment or taking responsibility for their own health.

Power

Look at Figure 2.1 again and think about *power*. The clinician is much more in control on the right-hand side, but this power slips away as the agenda increasingly becomes that of the patient. This is not to say that the patient-centred clinician does not have power. They simply have less direct control and are much less authoritarian. Patients historically expected and often wanted a powerful doctor; that is, a doctor who had reassuring authority, who is apparently capable and whose pronouncements can reduce anxiety. One definition of medical or "Aesculapian" authority divides it into three parts – *sapiential*, *moral*, and *charismatic*. These words are somewhat off-putting at first, but bear with us.

Sapiential Authority

This is the right to be heard based on knowledge or expertise, and it means that we must know, or at least appear to know, more about medicine than our patients. Medical knowledge is now much more freely available, thus reducing the intrinsic sapiential power of modern clinicians. Knowledge is often actively sought by our patients long before they reach the consultation. We are increasingly expected to confirm a diagnosis that a patient has already made (however erroneously) and are seen by patients as the enablers of investigations and treatment that the patient already knows (or thinks they know) they need. However, this is not universal; for some patients, sapiential authority can still be significant.

Moral Authority

This is the right to control and direct patients significantly, based on doing what society expects of us as clinicians. To retain our moral authority, we must always act with the good of the patient as our paramount concern (think of the Hippocratic Oath and, more recently, the General Medical Council's *Good Medical Practice*). This trust has been eroded in recent times due to multiple investigations into instances of poor care in hospitals, GP surgeries, and care homes, and high-profile court cases involving conflict over the treatment of very unwell children.

Charismatic Authority

This is the most difficult of the three concepts but boils down to many patients wanting clinicians to be a little magical. For most of us when we are ill, there is a need to supplement sapiential and moral authority with an ineffable factor, which might just hold out hope against the odds.

The three forms of authority are present in all of us, although the balance between them can vary significantly. For example, a partially patient-centred clinician has the same moral authority as their clinician-centred colleague, but they may reduce some of their sapiential authority by sharing more information with their patients. This highlights a fundamental truth. *Controlling information increases power and restricts patient involvement.* Many of us still feel very uneasy with knowledgeable and inquisitive patients, as such patients decrease our control. The partially patient-centred clinician will also be more likely to attempt to demystify the nature of medical diagnosis and treatment, reducing their charismatic authority and thus their power to control the interview. This requires a degree of bravery, particularly when first trying such strategies.

Control

Many of us are afraid of losing control. You may find yourself not asking the important questions due to a fear of opening an emotional Pandora's box and becoming overwhelmed; we use our power over our patient to keep the box shut and emotions at a non-threatening level. This style of behaviour can become fixed and persist throughout a career. Do not let this happen to you, or you will lose much more than you gain. Inevitably, the fear of losing control of the interaction is most acute at the beginning of your career. This is the time in your career when the need to appear to know more than your patient can easily make you appear dismissive and unempathic. It is inevitable that you will meet patients throughout your career who know more about their illness than you do. Can we reassure you now that admitting knowledge gaps is not the end of your authority? It may be the beginning of a truly therapeutic relationship, whether just in that one medical interaction or in a longer-term relationship.

We also know that patients often do not follow the advice we give them. The problem with the exercising of medical authority is that the overwhelming evidence suggests that *it is not very effective*. It quite obviously does not increase patient understanding. The often-quoted reason for this style of communication is that it will make patients do what is good for them, but it does not. As former US General Surgeon Dr C. Everett Koop said, "drugs don't work in patients who don't take them". There is an extensive body of literature looking at adherence to medical advice, summarised in NICE Clinical Guideline CG76, published in 2009 (and reviewed in 2015 when the evidence was found to be unchanged). This concludes that between a third and a half of all medication prescribed for a long-term condition is not taken as recommended. The term *compliance* with therapy, which implies a subservient or controlling relationship, is still commonly used, particularly in the context of us pronouncing patients "non-compliant". Instead, a better term is *concordance*, a negotiated, shared agreement between clinician and patient concerning treatment regimens, outcomes, and behaviours; a more cooperative relationship than those based on issues of compliance, non-compliance, and adherence.

These are the factors that can affect a clinician's agenda and the conscious or unconscious choices we make in our consultations based on agendas, power, and control. Now we need to look at the consultation from the patient's perspective to understand what matters to them. There are several methods to approach this concept and, as usual, it can be helpful to use a range of techniques when deciding what will work best for the patient in front of you.

The Health Belief Model

People's interest in their health and the degree to which they are motivated to change it – their health motivation – varies enormously. The health belief model (Alyafei et al.) is the most researched and validated description of patients' beliefs about health and related matters, and it has six main elements:

1. When considering specific health problems, people think very differently about how likely they are to be affected – their *perceived susceptibility*. For example, people who think that they are at high risk of developing lung cancer are more likely to follow advice about giving up smoking than those who do not think they are at risk. If a patient already has a health problem, their perceived vulnerability relates to the degree to which they believe in the diagnosis and its possible consequences. For example, suppose that a patient is diagnosed as having irritable bowel syndrome, and it is suggested that stress may be contributing to the condition. If the patient is convinced that bowel cancer and not stress is the cause, they are unlikely to adhere to the proposed management plan. This disbelief in what they are told may not be explicit and needs to be searched for.
2. Patients vary in how dire they believe the consequences of contracting a particular illness or of leaving it untreated would be – their *perceived severity*. Heart disease or lung cancer may seem to be a very remote possibility to a 16-year-old girl who is starting to smoke because of peer pressure. Her attitude may be: "And anyway, by the time I get to 40, they will have a cure for it, won't they?" Alternatively, the publicity about skin cancer resulting from sun exposure has meant that, in recent years, anxious patients have flocked to their GPs with a wide range of minor skin blemishes. Most people regard cancer as very serious, and some, if they suspect it, may even be too frightened to go to the doctor.
3. Patients may have very different perspectives on how beneficial the treatment or actions they are being asked to consider may be – the *perceived benefits*.
4. Balanced against the perceived benefits are the *perceived barriers* – patients weigh the advantages and disadvantages of taking a particular course of action. They do not necessarily take all the relevant considerations into account, but they make an evaluation nonetheless. This risk-benefit analysis is unique to each individual and can be influenced by others,

including us. However, to influence the equation, those factors that are already included by the patient need to be known. Thus, it becomes imperative for us to seek out such fears.

5 The fifth tenet of the health belief model has been added more recently, that of *self-efficacy*. This is a patient's belief, or the likelihood, of them being able to take the course of action proposed, be it dietary or lifestyle change, a course of treatment, or proposed medication.
6 Patients' beliefs do not already exist in a pre-packaged form. They are prompted or created by a number of stimuli and triggers – their *cues to action* – such as a physical sensation, what Granny said, what they read online, or what has just happened to the man down the road.

The health belief model emphasises what we already know. Patients are generally engaged in a struggle to understand what is happening to them, as well as what might happen. Different people try to resolve these dilemmas in different ways. Each person's belief system is of course unique, but it is strongly influenced by their upbringing, (sub)culture, and their immediate society. Searching for and acknowledging what matters to a patient is fundamental to understanding their beliefs.

Locus of Control

This is jargon for how we explain to ourselves what is likely to happen to our health. Using this idea, we can divide the human race into three types of people.

The Internal Controller

This type of person believes that fundamentally they are in charge of their own future health. In other words, what happens to their health is largely the result of their own actions. At one end of the scale, this is the health-conscious, vitamin-swallowing gym-goer who absorbs health-related news from papers, health blogs, social media, and online forums. (Most medical professionals are strong internal controllers.)

As far as communication is concerned, this type of person likes explanations and discussion; they want to be involved in decisions about their health, and they want to know what is happening. The medical arguments and explanations do not necessarily need to be rational; if the explanations are convincing, the internal controller will accept them.

The External Controller

This type of person is the opposite of the internal controller. They do not believe that they have any control over their health. What will be, will be. They are fatalists. External controllers are not keen on discussion, or at least not as far as their health is concerned. They want to be told what to do and then to ignore the advice or not as the case may be. They are not much into involvement and take little or no obvious interest in the media obsession with health matters. It is important for us to remember that the form of communication that will work best with the internal controller will not work well with the external controller. Now we come to the third type of person.

The Powerful Other

This type is quite different from the other two. They do not believe that they are in control of their own health, nor are they fatalists. They believe that *you* are in charge of their health. We see a disproportionate number of people of this variety. Many of those individuals who have been described as "heartsink" or "difficult" patients can be found in this category. A great many of these patients will have diagnosed, or more probably unacknowledged, mental health issues. The powerful others of this world pose another difficult challenge for us. Strategies that involve trying to give such patients more responsibility for their own health are often, at least initially, resisted. Getting them involved in deciding how to proceed is also difficult, as powerful others are quite firm about their agenda, and they are at their happiest with authoritarian clinicians who relieve them of any responsibility for their own health. They are not easily changed, and if their agenda for their health does not coincide with ours, they are unlikely to follow the medical advice that they are given.

As an example of a powerful other, imagine a middle-aged, obese patient with mild but symptomatic knee osteoarthritis, who utters the well-worn phrase "something must be done". As clinicians, we know that weight loss is likely to be effective in reducing her symptoms. However, your patient's perspective is that she wants relief from pain, a touch of medicinal magic, something fairly easy. She is well aware of her lifelong weight problem and certainly does not want the usual response she has heard since her twenties whenever she sees a doctor. She thinks that it is her clinician's responsibility to cure her pain, not hers. Your agendas are mismatched. This will remain a difficult consultation or series of consultations until one of you is prepared to change agendas. Can you do it? Should you?

As another example, imagine a young, health-anxious individual with a medical record already longer than average, mainly full of minor illnesses and over-investigated vague complaints. He presents feeling tired all the time and worried something is seriously wrong. You are not, and you try to reassure him, while discussing the impact of anxiety on physical health. You are almost certainly right, but you see him the next evening coming out of your colleague's surgery. Why? Perhaps because he wanted someone to take on board his fears, validate his symptoms, and diagnose a physical illness with a label. By contrast, you wanted to help the patient understand the psychological drive for his physical symptoms. What else might you have done? You could start by recognising his agenda, but more is needed to reach common ground.

Let's think about your agenda again. What do you want to achieve from the consultation and how are you going to do this? There are myriad strategies you could try, but which of them will work? What will satisfy you and yet help your patient?

Influencing Locus of Control

When Mrs Arthur first presented, she did not feel in control of the situation, nor was she fatalistic. She wanted you to take the lead, but she did expect a referral and an explanation. She could not be pigeonholed into any of the three categories described, but perhaps she is closest to a powerful other who, with support, involvement and some education, can be helped to take more control over her worrying illness.

The good thing about locus of control, as far as clinicians are concerned, is that it can be influenced.

Locus of control in most people is a tendency, not a fixed aspect of their personality. Think about your own beliefs and actions; are they always congruent with each other?

If it is correct that the communication strategy of the medical professional should be directed towards increasing people's tendency to look after and take some responsibility for their health – and we believe that it should – only the internal controllers are going to accept this idea easily. The others are going to need some persuading. However, the effort will be worthwhile for several reasons, not least because it is likely to lead to more patients following more medical advice.

If patients require different styles of communication depending on their locus of control, the key must be to explore our patients' agendas. If we know their ideas, concerns, and expectations, and we have an inkling about their locus of control, we can try to follow at least some, if not necessarily all, of their agenda, and talk to them about what matters to them and to us in ways that will engage them. Communication will become tailored to the individual and will therefore be more flexible and more effective, increasing the chances that our patient will actually follow our advice and get better or healthier.

When we think about trying to alter behaviours, linking lifestyle advice to a patient's individual health situation can be an effective tool (think of advising weight loss in the newly diagnosed type 2 diabetic); an intervention is much more likely to be effective if it is patient-centred and tailored to an individual's circumstances, attitudes, and choices.

In addition, think about the context in which we are seeing our patient; much like a patient's capacity, their beliefs, attitudes, and thoughts may vary in different scenarios. Think of a 30-year-old patient presenting with rectal bleeding; they may well think it is due to haemorrhoids. Now imagine their father died of bowel cancer; this probably changes their ideas and concerns. Or a patient with sensory symptoms which fit with meralgia paraesthetica, but who has a friend with advanced MS. Or a mother under stress with an unwell husband, who may not be able to be as rational about her poorly child as she would when life is easier.

Ideas, Concerns, and Expectations

Bearing all of this in mind, let's approach the concept of exploring a patient's ideas, concerns, and expectations again.

The best way to start is to imagine ourselves in the role of patient. After all, this is not too difficult; we have all been ill at some time and will be again. When people become ill, they ask themselves several questions, such as:

1. *What has happened?*
2. *Why has it happened?*
3. *Why has it happened to me?*
4. *Why now?*
5. *What should I do about it?*
6. *Should I go to the doctor?*

7 *Is it serious?*
8 *Can it be treated?*

Think of the last patient you saw. What questions do you think they had asked themselves? Imagine that last patient was you. What would you be asking yourself?

Let's return to the fictional Mrs Arthur from the beginning of this chapter. Suppose that we are now in the outpatient ENT clinic. The GP has stated in their referral that the thyroid function tests were borderline normal and that there is no family history of thyroid disease. In your detailed and systematic history taking, you have not discovered any symptoms referable to the thyroid gland, but the patient does seem to be rather anxious. Examination confirms a moderately enlarged gland with multiple small nodules; everything else is normal, but the patient seems to be slightly trembly and perhaps sweating more than you would expect. Now step aside from your history and examination and ask yourself what she might be thinking and feeling. Keep doing this.

Let us consider some of Mrs Arthur's possible thoughts and feelings. First, she is certainly frightened. Hospitals are terrifying places to most people. She is also afraid of the staff, especially the clinicians, *including you*. We can be frightening for several reasons; we tend to be dominant, powerful figures in the eyes of our patients, who have influence over their immediate and even long-term future. Mrs Arthur is also very concerned about herself. She has a lumpy enlargement in her neck, which to her is cancer until proved otherwise, and she will take a lot of convincing because her aunt died of cancer of the gullet (oesophagus to you) and she had lumps in her neck. She remembers the treatment was horrible and ineffective. She has vaguely heard about the thyroid gland and knows from a friend that one of the treatments is radioactive. This concerns her because she desperately wants children; she knows time is passing and she fears that a dose of radioactivity may put paid to her chances forever. She is afraid of having an operation because she has never been in hospital and hates the idea of being "put to sleep". She does not wish to lose control. She also knows from friends, the internet, and everyday experiences that operations can go wrong, and the neck seems to be a pretty dodgy place. Her husband produced a bundle of printouts from three websites he had found about the thyroid gland. She did not understand much of this information and could not bring herself to read some of the more alarming bits. She wishes that her husband was with her but worries that he has not really wanted to talk about her neck or her coming to the hospital. The bottom line is that she does not want to die.

The above description is only an imaginative guess at some of our patients' feelings, but how much of this did your history reveal, do you think?

As we have said, context is vital to understanding a patient's ICE. Not only do our past experiences colour our current thoughts, so does the situation in which we find ourselves at the time. As clinicians, we will have more medical insight than the average patient. Think about the last time you were ill. If you are always healthy, take a moment to get into role and imagine waking with a severe sore throat with a lot of swollen neck glands and feeling pretty ropey. Let's revisit the list of questions above:

1 *What has happened?* It's probably just a virus.
2 *Why has it happened?* I've been working late, I'm overtired, my resistance is a bit low.
3 *Why has it happened to me?* So annoying, but there's a lot going around.
4 *Why now?* Since Covid came along it always seems to be virus season.
5 *What should I do about it?* Dose myself up and it should just go away.
6 *Should I go to the doctor?* If it's viral, there's no point.
7 *Is it serious?* No, it will be getting better in a few days.
8 *Can it be treated?* There's no point in having antibiotics.

But what happens if your exams are two weeks away or you have a trip to Italy planned for next week?

1 *What has happened?* Oh no, maybe it is a streptococcus. I can't be ill now.
2 *What should I do about it?* I'd better get some antibiotics just in case. Maybe take some time off to nip it in the bud. Perhaps some zinc or vitamin C might help?
3 *Why has it happened to me?* I've been so busy, my immunity must be low. What if that bout of Covid did some immunological damage?
4 *Why now?* I can't believe this timing; it's the worst!
5 *What should I do about it?* I can't be ill now; I can't risk it; I need to try everything.
6 *Should I go to the doctor?* If I want to get antibiotics, I need to.
7 *Is it serious?* This might make me fail my exam. This will ruin my trip.
8 *Can it be treated?* I really hope so; I just can't afford to be ill now.

These questions and answers form the trinity of *ideas*, *concerns*, and *expectations.*

Now think about Mrs Arthur again and consider what sorts of things were going through her mind before she went to her GP for the first time. What she did *not* do was go to them with a multinodular goitre. She went because she had certain ideas about the lumpy swelling in her neck. She had several concerns and a few hazy expectations.

Nobody goes to a clinician with just a symptom. They go with *ideas* about the symptom, with *concerns* about the symptom and with *expectations* related to the symptom. Even in this modern age of endless quantities of information at our fingertips, and patients with much more detailed ideas, concerns, and expectations, this principle is unchanged.

Of course, the elephant in the room when discussing building therapeutic relationships with our patients through effective consulting is continuity of care. We fully recognise that the modern world of more transactional, fractured care delivery means that the continuity of the past, with hospital firms and list-holding GPs, is not the reality for many clinicians now. While the therapeutic benefit to patients of continuity of care with their clinician (particularly researched for GP interactions in the now-famous 2022 Norwegian study by Sandvik et al. published in the BJGP) is both experientially and research-proven to reduce morbidity and mortality, we know that many reading this book will not have the luxury of working in services that protect or promote continuity of care. As GPs who have been lucky enough to work in situations where continuity is prioritised, we believe strongly that this should be promoted at both a local and national level. But in the meantime, a lack of continuity means that every contact, every consultation needs to address a patient's ideas, concerns, and expectations.

Every consultation matters.

References

Alyafei A, Easton-Carr R. The Health Belief Model of Behavior Change. In: *StatPearls* [Internet]. Treasure Island, FL: StatPearls Publishing; 2025 Jan [updated 2024 May 19].

Sandvik H, Hetlevik Ø, Blinkenberg J, Hunskaar S. Continuity in general practice as predictor of mortality, acute hospitalisation, and use of out-of-hours care: a registry-based observational study in Norway. *Br J Gen Pract*. 2022;72(715): e84–e90.

CHAPTER

3 The Clinician and What Matters to Us

The single biggest problem in communication is the illusion that it has taken place.

Attributed to George Bernard Shaw

- What clinicians believe to be important in a consultation directly impacts how we conduct it.
- Understanding our own cognitive processing helps to understand common pitfalls in consulting.
- A lack of time or available resources does not limit our ability to improve the quality of our consultations.

In Chapter 2 we thought about the factors that affect patients' health understanding and decision-making. Let's now consider the role of clinicians; what factors influence how we consult? Understanding these enables us to be more effective.

Physical Health

How we feel affects how we consult. If you have a feverish cold and still find yourself at work, it can be very difficult to think straight and to make decisions. It is obvious that we consult better when we are well, but many of us,

DOI: 10.1201/9781003652137-3

driven by inner goals, continue long after the point when it would be better for our patients if we stopped. This needs to be recognised.

Emotional Health and Responses

Emotional health is subtler. The impact of our working environment, and the wider system around us, on our mental health cannot be overstated. Many UK hospitals and GP practices are understaffed and under-resourced. Morale is low, Covid was a traumatic nightmare for many, and demand from patients is high. Too many of us are focused on trying to cope with the day-to-day to have the time, or mental capacity, to look at the bigger picture, resulting in "burnout". Interest in patients as people wanes, their stories are not listened to, and their fears remain unexplored. If you feel yourself becoming emotionally stressed, acknowledge it, and try to seek help sooner rather than later. Roger Neighbour, in *The Inner Consultation* (2nd ed., 2005) discusses ways in which we can care for ourselves. He calls it "housekeeping", the point being that unless we can keep ourselves in good trim emotionally, we cease to be effective with our patients.

There is also the issue of how patients make us feel, and our response to that feeling. Michael Balint, a Hungarian psychoanalyst who founded the genuinely reflective "Balint Group", suggested that the way patients make us feel is a pretty good guide to how they are feeling (Balint, 1957). If we are able to recognise our own emotional responses to an interaction, this can tell us something profoundly useful about the person in front of us who provoked them. This is especially helpful when dealing with distressed patients who invoke strong responses in us. Understanding this process can help us avoid falling into roles the patient may unconsciously be making us adopt (acting like a parent, being overly punitive, crossing boundaries). It can also help us become more resilient to the impact of our patients' emotions, and less fearful of exploring them.

Dealing with people who are seeking your counsel can be immensely rewarding if you find that your knowledge and skills enable you to help them. This can give you an emotional high that is unmatched by most other occupations. However, there is a downside, too. You will meet many patients whom you cannot help very much, some in great distress. This will be hard, and you need to develop strategies to enable you to cope with this emotional pain. Helping someone to die peacefully can be gratifying if done well, especially with patients whom you have grown to know as people. There is the satisfaction of helping a fellow human being through those last days, weeks, or months, sharing knowledge, showing compassion, alleviating pain, facilitating communication with family, and not deserting them.

Attitudes and the "Medical Mind"

Like patients, we bring to our consultations a set of beliefs, moral values, and attitudes that are derived from our own upbringing, culture, and experience.

An excellent explanation of how attitudes affect our "medical mind" is contained in the 2011 book of the same name by Harvard physicians Professor Groopman and Dr Hartzband. These two married doctors reflect on their own differences in how they approach medical decisions, and how their varying backgrounds and upbringing have shaped this. They summarise three spectrums of belief which, combined, define our approach to medical decision-making. Groopman and Hartzband's work was derived from patient interviews, looking at how patients make medical decisions, but what is fascinating is that they also explore the clinician's "medical mind", recognising that the same principles apply to how clinicians approach medical decision-making. The first spectrum spans believers to doubters; believers will have faith in the power of medical intervention of all forms, while the doubters will approach any medical intervention with a large dose of scepticism. The second spectrum covers the range of beliefs from maximalists to minimalists; maximalists want to have all and every medical intervention available to them, while minimalists prefer to have the least medical interference possible. Finally, we have the spectrum from technologists to naturalists, with technologists wanting to utilise the latest medical technologies, while naturalists prefer the most natural, non-medical approach possible. Putting all this together, we are able to group our patients into decision-making cohorts, much as we discussed in the last chapter with locus of control. For example, the maximalist, technological, believer will jump on the offer of a statin at a QRISK of 11%, while the minimalist, natural, doubter wouldn't touch it with a bargepole. However, we can also apply this to ourselves as clinicians. What is your true attitude to QRISK and risk-based preventative approaches? As a clinician are you a believer or a doubter, a maximalist or a minimalist, and a technologist or a naturalist? Where you fall on these spectrums will undoubtedly impact how you consult with your patients, which ones you find it easy to come to a shared decision with, and which patients challenge you the most.

The point we wish to make about attitudes is that they govern our behaviour, both ours and our patients'. People's attitudes are not necessarily what they say they are. Previous MRCGP exam candidates have demonstrated this aptly; when claiming to believe in and practise the patient-centred method, video recordings of actual consultations submitted for the old video MRCGP exam showed only 10% of candidates actually did. Their stated attitudes did not lead to the relevant behaviour, so the attitude must not be the real one. Think about your attitudes to patients and communicating and be honest with yourself, what is your real attitude? Think about your own beliefs and attitudes. Can you compromise from time to time? Can you justify your attitudes to yourself or to your peers? Our self-esteem is also relevant here. We all want to be liked, and wanting to be liked by our patients can be dangerous. A clinician who always pleases their patient and never receives complaints is likely to be avoiding the difficult conversations.

Motivation is probably the key. We will not communicate well with patients or anyone else if we lack the motivation to do so. Exams are an excellent motivator, of course. If communication must be demonstrated to pass, we learn how to do it, even if it does not come naturally to us. Once they are over, however, we can do as we like. And if communication was not something we believed to be important day-to-day, then our motivation will fall and so will our effectiveness. Good communication is effortful, and as other demands creep in it can fall down the priority list. Practising patient-centred medicine is in fact pretty easy if you want to do it; you just have to listen, be curious, and participate in a dialogue rather than a monologue, but you do have to *want* to do it. If you do not, why not? Changes in doctor behaviour in this regard over the years have been shown to be agonisingly slow, presumably because the majority still do not regard patient-centred, evidence-based, shared decision-making as worth the time and emotional effort to them, and if they feel like that, all of the knowledgeable and clever teaching in the world is going to make very little difference. So, the first step towards improving your communication skills is to get your attitude right. Professor Roger Kneebone provides a novel interpretation of this by drawing parallels between the close-up, live performances of magic and medicine in his article "Performing Magic, Performing Medicine":

> *By framing the clinical consultation as a close-up live performance with a very small audience, the focus shifts from the acquisition and application of scientific knowledge (an internal focus of attention) to an encounter where a narrative is jointly constructed and where the patient's perspective is prime (an external focus of attention).*

Empathy

As you will hopefully now be appreciating, good consulting skills require effort. The same goes for empathy. Many clinicians will espouse being good at empathy, but true empathy, much like exploring ICE, is so much more than a box-ticking exercise. The idea is to identify mentally with the patient and so fully comprehend them. However, in many scenarios true empathy is challenging. For example, can middle-class clinicians really empathise with someone caught up in substance misuse and petty crime? We can be compassionate, and we can care for them, but the majority will be unable to truly empathise. Empathy is about *trying to understand*. We might not succeed, but we should make the effort to try to imagine their situation in order to communicate effectively with them.

Remember Mrs Arthur from the last chapter with her ideas, concerns, and expectations. This first example from the ENT outpatients is of the clinician making all the right noises, but without any effort to be truly empathic.

> Mrs Arthur … Don't worry about the thyroid gland, we will get it sorted for you … are you having a holiday this year? [while typing up blood test requests on the computer] … I bet your husband is worried about you [still filling in the form, and paying no attention to her response] … Well, now, off you go and get these tests done – we will see you with the results soon and then fix the right treatment for you. It has been really nice to meet you, and you mustn't worry about anything.

This second example shows genuine empathy and demonstrates the skill of the clinician who is actively showing a desire to truly understand Mrs Arthur's feelings.

> Hello, Mrs Arthur, you have finally made it to clinic, so what has been on your mind? … Is that what you were worried about? Cancer like your aunt? I can see why that would have been a concern for you, but I don't think that's what's going on – but you are in the right place for us to make the correct diagnosis and give you the right treatment … What do you know about the thyroid gland? … We may have to give you some radiation treatment with a special iodine. How do you feel about that? … I don't think that is a risk to you getting pregnant in the future, but I hear how important starting a family is to you. I will find out more details from my registrar and get back to you.

Next time we can go through some of your worries ... What are you going to tell your husband about what we have discussed? ... Ah, it sounds like he's very worried about you. Take this leaflet home; you can give it to him to read so he understands what's going on ... See you in a month, and have a good holiday. In the meantime, you really don't need to let this prey on your mind ... Yes, goodbye then [turns to computer to start requesting investigations].

Does empathy matter? Absolutely. David Loxterkamp's essay in the BMJ in 2008, although now over 15 years old, eloquently explains why.

When a patient visits the doctor, he or she hopes to be reassured that the lump is not cancer; that the pain will soon end; that a ladder leads from this despair ... If all of this could be accomplished with computerised interviews, health maintenance check-lists and evidence-based guidelines, we would not need doctors. Vulnerable patients come to us in desperation. Their fears and insecurities must be met with authority, knowledge and action. But their humanity requires something more: a handshake, a funny story, our undivided attention – and all that this implies: a doctor who will champion and remain faithful to their cause.

Intuition, Perceptiveness, and Experience

Intuitive medical behaviour may be based on experience – effectively a synaptic short-circuit – but some doctors are better at it than others. Usually, the more intuitive doctors are the more experienced ones. When you are learning, do not trust too much to intuition. Go back, recheck, and try to trace the intuitive pathway until you can follow the logical thread.

Expert intuition is often akin to a simple algorithm, although it can be better than this if steered in a structured direction to consider all the relevant information. We must avoid "what you see is all there is" or, in other words, making hasty decisions based only on the obvious information in front of us without searching for all the other relevant factors. Daniel Kahneman's excellent 2011 book *Thinking, Fast and Slow* explains this in more detail, and we would highly recommend this eye-opening insight into how our brains make decisions.

System 1 and System 2 are metaphors Kahneman uses for our different cognitive-processing abilities. System 1 is our automatic brain, which offers up information it feels is relevant and associated with the issue at hand, without any effort on our part; the intuition-generator. Our System 1 offers us this even when the evidence it is based on is incomplete or inaccurate. We do not choose to experience an emotional reaction or a perception; they just happen. System 2 is conscious and effortful and has the role of endorsing or discarding the information presented to it by System 1. We have a limited capacity for effortful thinking; most of us cannot solve a complex puzzle while negotiating a busy roundabout. *Thinking about a patient's unconscious communication requires effort.* We perform better at tasks requiring System 2 input when we have adequate glucose, are not distracted, take time, and are frowning (yes, really!). Perceptiveness is a System 2 process; it is effortful and must be learned. Remember, Sherlock Holmes, one of the finest role models of intuition and perceptiveness, was based by Conan Doyle on a senior medical professional of the time in Edinburgh.

If our patient gets better because of our decisions, this feeds back into our knowledge store, as does the patient who does not get better. We live in the rapidly increasing world of evidence-based medicine, but most will still trust our own experience of ten people on a particular drug more than a clinical trial of 1,000 patients. This is not to deride the scientific basis of some of our knowledge or to belittle the power of the double-blind randomised controlled trial (though we discuss the biases and limitations of medical evidence in Chapter 8), but to acknowledge human behaviour and the power of personal experience. This is the concept of *cognitive ease*, where we are more likely to make a decision based on something we can easily recall, such as a recent patient's successful outcome, than search through our memory banks for another solution, such as the data from the latest trial. Conversely, our previous experience can make a huge difference to the way we consult in the future – once you have seen one aggressive glioblastoma presenting as a headache, or motor neurone disease presenting as a simple, mechanical-sounding fall, it is hard not to be reminded of them in future, similar presentations. Some academics deride our humanistic "evidence", which typically focuses on outcomes in small numbers of patients, as they point out that such small samples cannot possibly be statistically significant, however much we might want to see a pattern emerging. *But* the story that makes more sense to us will seem overwhelmingly more appealing. How plausible and how likely something is are completely different but easily confused concepts. Our System 2s require effort and often fail to apply the correct rule unless we force ourselves to examine our thinking critically.

Every patient is unique, and this is why medicine is so difficult to teach and to learn. What works for one patient will not work for another. If we observe the outcomes carefully and develop our perception, this will feed back into both our knowledge and our understanding store and will increase our intuitiveness. Consulting with and examining patients forms the structure for developing your intuition and perceptive skills. Really seeing them, truly hearing what they say (or do not say) and understanding them and their context are the flesh on those bones.

External Limitations and Continuity

We fully admit it is not quick or easy to consult well, and this is exacerbated by the environment in which many of us find ourselves working. Target-driven, guideline- and protocol-led defensive medical practice at a time of workload and workforce crises creates a perfect storm for burnout and disengagement. However, you must try hard not to let this put you off. Great communication is always possible, even within extremely short patient interactions in corridors and surrounded by chaos, if you use your skills to produce effective communication.

As we touched on in the previous chapter, the loss of continuity of care has not only had an impact on a patient's experience and outcome, but on our ability to consult effectively. This is particularly relevant in UK general practice, where continuity of care leads to the development of a medical relationship over an extended timeframe, the model which many longer-serving GPs remember and lament the loss of. The UK system of general practice used to be an international benchmark of high-quality, low-cost healthcare centred on longitudinal relationship-based medicine, but this is in sharp decline. For those of us who have had the opportunity to experience continuity with our patients, we know the value of it. Difficult conversations become so much easier when trust has already been earned and established. Patients are more likely to follow our advice because they know it worked last time, and so they have confidence it will again. Patients also much better understand the thorny issues of medical uncertainty when discussed with a trusted clinician, and they more easily accept the fact that sometimes we are not right and we will make the wrong treatment choices, or a mistake, because they know us as people and individuals in our own right. For us as clinicians, there are obvious benefits; we already know our patients, we are not having to establish a new rapport and relationship in every consult, and we can use our previously learned knowledge of a patient's situation, background, and medical history alongside their previously elicited ideas, concerns, and expectations. This does not mean we should not make the effort to explore these with each new presentation; on the contrary, patients have an excellent tendency to surprise us with a completely different decision or perspective to the one we predicted. However, in the majority, that prior knowledge will save us time without losing the essence of what matters. It is the understanding of this complexity of human decision-making that brings us back to the importance of really working out what matters, and continuity is such a powerful tool. Remember the Norwegian study we mentioned in the last chapter; Sandvik et al. have shown that length of continuity with a named GP is significantly associated with lower use of out-of-hours services, fewer acute hospital admissions, and lower mortality. In addition, they confirmed the presence of a causal dose-response relationship, which means that the longer the continuity with the same GP, the greater the benefits seen. Imagine if this level of benefit was seen with a new drug or treatment; it would be on newspaper front pages as the new miracle cure.

So, what is the result of this insight into how our brains tick as clinicians? It is the recognition that if we can try to approach each consultation with an open and enquiring mind, an attitude to want to genuinely learn about the patient in front of us, to understand what matters to them, their ideas, concerns, and expectations, and an appreciation of the knowledge, experience, and intuition that drives us, we will be well on the way to having an effective consultation with that patient. If we can attempt to do all of this while appreciating that the environment we are working in may not be ideal, or even particularly conducive to achieving it, yet we understand why it is important to try anyway, we will without a doubt make more of a difference to the patient sitting in front of us than if we didn't. Every experience will add to our store of knowledge, and each one is an opportunity to try to achieve a genuine shared understanding, testing out different techniques, and adapting to each patient as an individual. Over time we will reap the rewards of effective communication and understanding, whether through developing trust in a therapeutic relationship, or simply being more likely to reach a shared decision and treatment plan that our patients are more likely to understand, agree with, and therefore follow. Surely that is what really matters to us.

References

Balint M. *The Doctor, his Patient and the Illness*. London: Tavistock Publications; 1957.

Groopman J and Hartzband P. *Our medical mind: how to decide what is right for you*. Penguin Press; 2011.

Kahneman D. *Thinking, Fast and Slow*. New York: Farrar, Straus and Giroux; 2011.

Kneebone RL. Performing magic, performing medicine. *Lancet*. 2017;389:148–149.

Loxterkamp D. Why rivers run: On the headwaters of family medicine. *BMJ*. 2008;337:a2575.

Neighbour R. *The Inner Consultation*. 2nd ed. Oxford: Radcliffe Publishing; 2005.
Sandvik H, Hetlevik Ø, Blinkenberg J, Hunskaar S. Continuity in general practice as predictor of mortality, acute hospitalisation, and use of out-of-hours care: a registry-based observational study in Norway. *Br J Gen Pract*. 2022;72(715):e84–e90.

CHAPTER 4

Technique Matters

The most important thing in communication is hearing what isn't said.

Peter Drucker

- Ideas, concerns, and expectations exist in layers, guarded by different degrees of reticence.
- Exploring them won't feel awkward once their common origins are understood.
- Actively listening clinicians pick up cues to ICE at any point during a consultation.

When Peter first began promulgating the concept of ICE in the 1990s, its application was purely in postgraduate training for GPs. Over the course of a generation, however, it has become widely disseminated. ICE is now introduced from the outset in most medical schools, and proponents of truly patient-centred consulting can be found in every speciality and branch of medical practice.

Yet although the understanding that patients' ideas, concerns, and expectations are central to effective consulting is now widespread, training in how to elicit ICE has lagged woefully behind. Clinicians at the beginning of their careers are commonly taught to ask questions such as "What do you think is

DOI: 10.1201/9781003652137-4

going on?" or "What do you expect me to do?". While commendably direct, such prompts frequently backfire. Perplexed patients, rightly expecting to be consulting with someone with more than a smidgeon of "Aesculapian" medical authority, often misinterpret such questions as indicating cluelessness in their clinician instead. How often do such well-meant but clumsy enquiries result in a surprised look on a patient's face and the nonplussed response: "Well, you're the doctor!"? Even worse, clunkily phrased ICE questions are frequently misinterpreted by understandably anxious patients as dismissive.

We suspect that these awkward outcomes are one factor behind many clinicians' reluctance to explore ICE thoroughly. It becomes a potentially embarrassing task or chore to be got through as quickly as possible, a box to be ticked and swiftly moved on from. The patient with tension headache? ICE, brain tumour – check! The patient with costochondritis? ICE, heart attack – check! While these are undoubtedly important ideas to address, they are highly likely to be superficial and incomplete. Merely the tip, we might say, of the ICEberg.

So how do we go about eliciting our patients' ICE in more natural, meaningful ways? In Chapter 2, we saw that no one goes to a clinician with a symptom; they go with ideas, concerns, and expectations about their symptom, and they are engaged in a struggle to understand what it means for them. Those ideas, concerns, and expectations arise from two things: that unique patient's *knowledge* and their personal *context*.

Knowledge

Knowledge is chiefly derived from a limited set of sources. For most people, it will be based on things they have *read* (these days, almost exclusively online and increasingly the output of large language models like ChatGPT or Claude, but it could be magazine or newspaper articles, or books they have come across); things they have *heard* (usually what family and close friends tell them, but sometimes work colleagues or that bloke down the pub, or an interview with a celebrity on the radio); things they have *watched* (often videos pushed into their feed by obliging social media algorithms, but documentaries are another source); and things they have *experienced* (previous illness themselves or with someone they know, including how clinicians have behaved in the past).

Armed with this appreciation, we can open ICE discussions in much more subtle ways. There are myriad approaches, but consider the following examples:

These days, most people research their symptoms online. What have you been finding out?

What do your family or friends think about it all?

Have you had anything like this before, or know anyone who has?

These kinds of questions are genuinely *curious*, opening the door for patients to contribute to the conversation, as well as communicating our interest in what they have to say without the risk of appearing professionally inept. Try them out and see how you get on.

Context

The same symptom or disease will mean completely different things for each patient. Knee pain in a septuagenarian might be disturbing their sleep, and their spouse's too. For a keen athlete, it might threaten their ability to compete in the next championships. Diarrhoea might be causing a data analyst to take embarrassingly frequent loo breaks at work; to a forty-something single parent, it might herald the bowel cancer that could leave their children orphaned.

Again, there are innumerable ways to explore context, but consider the following examples:

That sounds difficult. How is it affecting your daily life?

I can see this must be worrying. What do you worry about most?

Reticence, Layers, Cues, and Active Listening

These example questions are all "open", initiating conversation rather than requiring yes/no responses. Sometimes they will yield immediate results, and your patient will need no further invitation to contribute. Indeed, as ICE has permeated throughout the medical world, so many patients have learned (or been "trained") that clinicians want to understand their agenda and will come prepared to explain their perspectives (indeed, you will sometimes encounter patients nowadays who will lay out their ICE unprompted at the start of a consultation).

But a common mistake is to assume that everything worth knowing will readily flow. More usually, people's ICE exists in *layers* and there are variable degrees of *reticence* about verbalising them.

Think back to the scenario in Chapter 2 where you've been struck down by a sore throat and decide to attend your GP practice. If invited, you're more than happy to explain how it's so painful you can hardly swallow and that you're not sleeping well. You might be equally comfortable explaining you've got an important exam in a couple of weeks' time. Maybe, though, you wouldn't be so forthcoming about your anxiety if it's a holiday to Italy you're worried about – that might feel a more self-indulgent reason to have taken up NHS time. And what you're really hoping for is a course of antibiotics, but you are almost certainly not going to disclose that. You think it would be rude if you seem to be telling a colleague how to do their job, or you might feel ashamed because you know that the medically "right" approach would be to allow it the chance to self-limit for four or five days and you fear they will think badly of you. As to those niggling concerns in the far back of your mind – that the bouts of Covid you've had might have damaged your immune system in some way ... well, you're sure your colleague would laugh at you, or think you're a hypochondriac or something.

Furthermore, not infrequently the deepest layers of ICE lie in the subconscious and we are not immediately aware of them. Maybe it would only be when the clinician asks if you know anyone else who's had recurrent sore throats that it triggers the memory of your friend in sixth form who kept being off with tonsillitis in the months before his non-Hodgkin's lymphoma first presented.

While this example scenario stars you, a clinically trained healthcare professional, exactly the same themes apply to patients from every walk of life, though the power imbalances discussed in earlier chapters make it even more likely that reticence will prevent the more personal or potentially embarrassing layers of ICE from being articulated.

How then, if ICE is so multilayered and often well guarded, do we go about exploring it all? This is where good consultation skills are vital. Remember that the majority of human communication happens non-verbally – through eye contact or lack of it; via body posture and gesture. Beyond the actual words we choose, we articulate far more in the rate and volume of our speech; by the pauses, repetitions, non-sequiturs, similes, and metaphors we employ; and often by what we don't say.

This is where *active listening* is so important. Even though a patient's ICE will often be multilayered and variably inaccessible, they will usually communicate important things non-verbally. Active listening involves consciously attending to the totality of someone's communication, with particular emphasis on the non-verbal, seeking out the *cues* that tell us more than the words they're saying. This might be an aversion of gaze, a sudden folding of arms, a long pause before replying. Watch for "consultation tennis", where a patient raises the same point two or more times (like batting a ball back over the net at you), telling you there's something you haven't addressed. Or non-sequiturs, a response that doesn't follow from what's just been said, suggesting that a chain of thought has just gone through their mind. There are innumerable examples, and we give more detail in the Appendix. The key point is to expect that cues will arise, practise looking out for them, and when you notice them, reflect them back in open form to encourage exploration: "You seemed upset there", "You've mentioned being off your food a couple of times", "You described your headache as like a pressure". Then see where things take you.

One final point. The incorporation of ICE into the traditional clerking model with its own "slot" (PC, HPC, PMH, DH, SOH, ICE, etc.), and consultation tools such as Damian Kenny's otherwise excellent "Crossing the Bridge", creates the impression that eliciting ICE belongs only to one specific, early part of the consultation. It does not. Patients will give you cues at any time: during or after an examination, for example; even when their hand is on the door handle on the way out. Indeed, the most guarded and often the most significant aspects of ICE will only be disclosed once rapport has been built and the patient has finally decided they can trust you. Keep your active listening ears tuned in at all times.

Both the types of thinking we met in Chapter 3, Kahneman's System 1 and System 2, are important to active listening. Often, you'll be struck by intuitions, so listen to them. But non-verbal communication and cues will frequently pass us by unless we're engaging System 2 and consciously thinking about what a patient is really telling us. And pay attention to how a consultation is making you feel; as discussed earlier, this can give important insights into your patient's emotional state.

Once you have the fullest picture possible of your patient's ICE, you are in pole position to arrive at a shared understanding and plan with them. Your septuagenarian with knee pain might be happy with some nocturnal analgesia, your amateur athlete might be better connected with a sports physio. Your data analyst might be helped by some loperamide while their gastroenteritis settles, your single parent might only be at peace after a negative FIT.

The skills outlined in this chapter take time and experience to learn and become proficient in. In the early stages of our careers, where much of our brain power is preoccupied with trying to make sense of things medically – arriving at a diagnosis or deciding what to do – there is little cognitive bandwidth available for active listening. As the more biomedical aspects of our role become second nature, we find we can devote more of our attention to the nuances of interpersonal communication. But don't park these matters in a space labelled "for another day". Effortful as it is, keep trying to incorporate active listening into your practice from the outset: it will soon get easier as a result. The consultation style we establish early in our careers tends to become our default, and difficult to change later. Make yours patient-centred, and your medical encounters will be immeasurably better for it, as will the experiences of the patients you care for.

References

Kahneman D. *Thinking, Fast and Slow*. New York: Farrar, Straus and Giroux; 2011.
Moyers B. *A World of Ideas*. Interview; 1989.

CHAPTER

5

The Consultation – What Truly Matters

Sometimes, the best thing we can do for our patients is to tell them what the best behaviour is and then negotiate something they can live with.

Nancy Dickey

- Effective communication is more likely to lead to behaviour change.
- A patient's experiences are fundamental to their health beliefs; exploring these is key.
- Understanding availability and confirmation biases is important for both patient and clinician.

We have looked at the patient and clinician factors that are needed to achieve an effective, meaningful consultation, and some techniques for doing so. But how do we measure success or achievement? We can glean this from looking at the possible outcomes of the consultation. These can be divided into immediate, intermediate, and long term.

Immediate Outcomes

It is for our knowledge, and the skills in applying that knowledge, that the public come to us. We have seen that we need to strive to achieve more than

DOI: 10.1201/9781003652137-5

just the imparting of medical wisdom to produce a genuine understanding, a commitment to plan, and potentially a change in behaviour in our patients. During an effective consultation, a relationship will have been formed, the beginning of trust.

Commitment to Plan

After a patient has consulted you, they make an immediate decision whether to follow your advice, and there are many reasons why they may do so. The first and best is that they believe and understand you, and their agenda approximates yours closely. Or it may be doing what one is told by a respected professional. It is important to note that patients are more likely to follow your advice if they like you, because they are much more likely to see you as trustworthy and wise. Remember continuity of care, the respect and trust your patients need to develop a trusting relationship – this is much more likely to happen when they have the chance to get to know you. As already discussed, many studies have proven the beneficial impact of continuity of care in general practice. A systematic review in the BMJ (Pereira Gray et al., 2018) looked at continuity of care and demonstrated that increased continuity with a doctor was associated with lower patient mortality rates; the more often a patient sees the same doctor, the more likely they are to form an effective therapeutic relationship. This was found to apply to both generalist and specialist doctors and highlights the vital importance of continuity in today's ever-fragmenting health service.

There is also commitment from us as clinicians. We cannot commit ourselves deeply to every patient with whom we come into contact, or we would be swamped (see Roger Neighbour's The Inner Consultation). However, we must give each of our patients a degree of commitment, and for some, this will be more than others. Think of the palliative paediatric patient to whose parents you give your mobile number for them to contact you out of hours, in contrast to the patients in whom we are trying to reduce over-reliance on appointments and our input. It is part of our learning to judge the appropriate level of commitment that we need to make to an individual who seeks our help.

Change of Concern and Behaviour

The immediate thought most of us have is that consulting with us will reduce our patients' concern. This is often not true of course. Let us take three patients with a headache as an example.

The first patient is a 25-year-old woman who is afraid of her recurrent headaches and thinks that she probably has a brain tumour. She is hoping to be taken seriously and properly investigated and treated. It is you who are due to see her, and you are rushed. Although you do not discover all her story, you do discover her fear of a brain tumour and see her immense relief at being allowed to talk about it. You examine her thoroughly, including her fundi, which is, of course, intended to be both diagnostic and therapeutic. After discussion, explanation, advice, and the offer of a possible follow-up appointment, she leaves you with less concern than when she arrived. Her health understanding has changed a little, although we know this may not last.

Your second patient is a 56-year-old banker who says that he is not too concerned about his recent onset of migraines because his mother got them at about this age, but he would like some of those new injections which he read about on the internet. You go through the same routine, but the headaches don't sound typical of migraine and are waking him from sleep, prompting an urgent neurological referral. He is grateful but worried. This illustrates the rather obvious point that concern can increase after a successful consultation.

Your third patient is a 48-year-old lady who is perimenopausal and experiencing a worsening of her known migraines. She has read about the various prophylactic medication options but is very worried about potential side effects. You are having a bad day and fail to pick up on the cues, instead telling her that you think beta-blockers would be a good place to start. You give her an entirely appropriate prescription, but as nothing you have said has alleviated her concerns, her health understanding remains unchanged, and she is unlikely to take the medication.

The effect that the clinician's style can have on the patient's concern is worth repeating. Respected authoritarian clinicians have the power to reduce anxiety but at the cost of reducing patient autonomy. However, giving ill patients too much autonomy can make a clinician appear indecisive or uncertain, increasing anxiety. This is a difficult balance to get right, but it does warrant trying. Sharing information and understanding is most likely to increase autonomy while constraining any increase in anxiety.

The last point about concern relates to a well-known graph: a simple but very important curve (Figure 5.1).

As you can see, performance increases with concern up to a certain point, then plateaus and falls off. This curve should interest us because it demonstrates that if their anxiety or concern is too great, patients will not do what

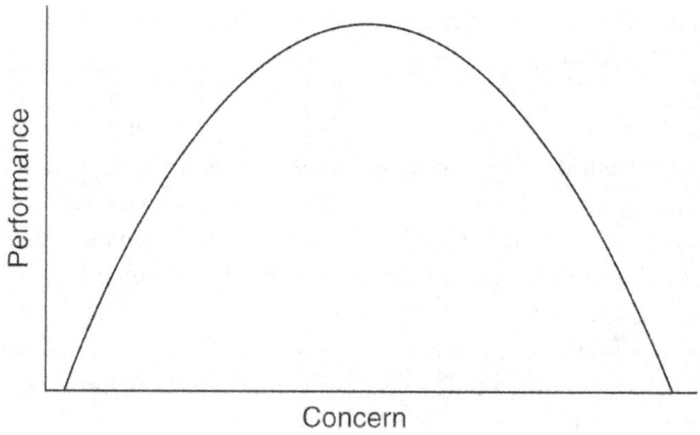

FIGURE 5.1 Concern measured against performance.

is in their best interests. This may be why the scare tactic of showing graphic images on cigarette packets is not usually a very effective technique for helping smokers to give up; it pushes the majority over the top of the curve. Too great a fear of cancer freezes patients into inertia and usually also stops them from hearing what you are saying. But a small decrease in concern may put them on peak performance to enable them to feel empowered to change. We have all been taught about the change cycle and its phases of precontemplation, contemplation, changing behaviour, maintaining behaviour, and for many, relapsing. It is also true that people must be in the right frame of mind to change their health behaviour, and your input at the right time can be crucial.

Satisfaction

The simple perspective here is that high patient satisfaction is good, and low patient satisfaction is bad. However, as usual, life is not quite that straightforward. Many health promotion messages are not particularly satisfying for patients, even if they are based on good evidence. However, in addition to the importance of proactive health prevention strategies, as GP payments are linked to lifestyle change measures such as smoking cessation, weight management referrals, cervical screening, and immunisation; this becomes a necessary part of every consultation in general practice. The patient comes with a cough and is told to stop smoking, lose weight, have a cervical smear, and is then told that she cannot have any antibiotics prescribed. To a large proportion of our patients this may be profoundly unsatisfying, but to most of us this is engaging with preventative medicine, as well as being essential for a GP practice's financial survival.

There is an easy way to satisfy most patients, and that is to give them what they want, but the fact that patients often want treatments such as unnecessary antibiotics, excessive time, more of you than you can spare, dubious operations, and so on means that the goal of only satisfying patients is a poor one. We need more integrity than that. But it does seem that satisfying our patients is important because evidence shows that satisfied patients are more likely to follow medical advice (Little et al., 2001). There is little evidence that time makes much difference, but communication and style do. It seems to be the case that warm, friendly doctors are more likely to satisfy patients than cold, business-like ones. In the jargon, "positive affect" works well. It also appears that doctors talking too much reduces satisfaction, whereas the sense of being listened to and understood increases it. Therefore, quite simply, patients like doctors who smile at them, are friendly, positive, and actively listen to them, and within this framework they will then accept some of the less pleasant health messages.

We also need to consider the clinician's satisfaction with a consultation. We all want to do a good job and to take pride in doing so. This affects how we perform. For instance, there is some evidence that doctors who have low job satisfaction prescribe more tranquillisers and antibiotics and have shorter consultations. These days, job satisfaction is sadly becoming more of a rarity. To derive regular satisfaction from patient encounters, we need to like what we are doing, have reasonably clearly defined aims, and obtain frequent, supportive feedback that tells us how we are doing and how we can improve. We suspect that not many of us receive much of that type of feedback from either our patients or our peers, both in hospital and general practice. It is difficult to feel satisfaction when you never know whether what you are doing is of any use, and you rarely see patients get better as a result of something you have done. This brings us back once again to continuity of care, and recognising the value of continuity for clinicians, as well as our patients.

Feedback

It is worth thinking further about feedback for a minute. The feedback that we receive from our patients is haphazard and highly selective. The happy ones come back, write us letters, send us occasional presents, tell us how good we are and make us feel good about ourselves. The patients with whom we have been less successful may never come back. They probably will not contact us at all, although a few will complain. This means that feedback from patients is polarised and can be distorted in our favour. Clinicians need unbiased, constructive feedback. The use of patient satisfaction questionnaires is going some way towards improving this situation, but most of the feedback is general, whereas it is the specific feedback that we find most useful. In this modern age of increasing numbers of patient feedback options, particularly online reviews, some use them in the spirit in which they were intended, but often these reviews are given anonymously, and they can be vicious, with no real way for those reviewed to challenge or refute what may feel unfair or unfounded criticisms. Social media can be kind but is often very hurtful and impossible to respond to. Recognise the importance of how this makes you feel, and the impact this has on your work.

Intermediate Outcomes

Concordance

There is a difference between a patient's commitment to a plan and immediate thoughts or plans to follow it, to the full follow-through to complete the plan. Dropping out or losing momentum can occur at any stage. However, we already know that our patient is more likely to follow their treatment if they understand and believe the explanation. Some patients will do it simply because they have been told to. But most will follow it if their own understanding seems to match that of the clinician and their agenda is shared – this is what is meant by concordance.

Concordance is a fascinating area that we know very little about from our experiences with patients – we rarely hear what lessons our patients learn from whether they follow our advice or not. Around 99% of patients act rationally in terms of their own health beliefs which, however, may not themselves be rational. In Table 5.1, let's imagine various outcomes for a patient following a consultation with a sore throat where the treatment given was antibiotics.

Patient A wants penicillin for her sore throat. She is given the antibiotic, gets better, and has her health belief confirmed, that penicillin cures sore throats. She is highly likely to consult with the same problem when it arises again, often at the first onset of symptoms.

Patient B does exactly the same thing but does not get better. What lessons has he learned? That penicillin does not cure sore throats? That it was not

TABLE 5.1 The Effect of Adherence on Understanding

	Patient gets well	Patient does not get well
Patient adheres to treatment	A	B
Patient does not adhere to treatment	C	D

a "strong" enough antibiotic ("I've always had the green ones before; these red ones are useless")? That the clinician was right all the time and it was a virus that did not respond to penicillin? That there may be something very serious which was missed? That this clinician is no good and that he will try a different one next time? And so on.

What about Patient C? He only came for a sick note but was given tablets that he did not want and did not take, and he got better anyway.

Or what about Patient D? She was given penicillin but did not take it because it had given her thrush last time. Now she feels both unwell and guilty. If she goes back to the doctor she might well lie about taking the tablets.

These are just some examples of the types of messages that our patients get from whether they do or do not take our advice. How many of these are we aware of? Our patients' health understanding will be changed by a combination of each consultation *and* by the outcomes of those consultations.

Knowledge and Understanding

A major stumbling block in establishing shared understanding between clinicians and patients concerns our different frames of reference. Clinicians are taught scientifically, learn thousands of complicated words, and have models of disease imprinted in their brains. Patients are not like this. This disparity can significantly differ depending on the type of consultation in question; an acute illness such as a sore throat provides a clearly discrete episode with fairly binary outcomes as above. However, the management of a long-term condition provides more opportunities for explanation and education with our patients, allowing us to develop their medical understanding, which is usually helpful in improving concordance and behaviour change.

When we consider the development of understanding, it is important to return again to Daniel Kahneman's *Thinking, Fast and Slow* (2011). Kahneman describes our inbuilt tendency to jump to conclusions and then to look for the facts that will confirm these opinions. He calls this *confirmation bias*. Clinicians often do this without thinking when we make a diagnosis; we must actively force ourselves to consider other possibilities. Patients do this too; during a conversation with you they may receive a message that you may or may not have meant, but in the subsequent dialogue and after leaving the consultation they will continue to search for the evidence that confirms their initial conclusion. Most of us seek data that are compatible with the beliefs we already hold, and to do otherwise requires conscious effort on our part.

A related concept is that of *availability bias*, another mental shortcut where we overestimate the likelihood of an event or explanation based on examples that come easily to mind – we tend to rely on vivid or recent memories rather than objective statistics. Think how differently you might approach a woman with non-specific abdominal pain if the last such patient, after several inconclusive consultations, transpired to have ovarian cancer. Patients, too, are susceptible to availability bias and as the medical journalist Deborah Cohen describes in her book *Bad Influence* (Cohen, 2026), it is an increasingly important factor in the social media age. The minute we show interest in a particular health issue online, the algorithms running in the background will start pushing related content into our feed. Click "like" on a video about one woman's ovarian cancer experience and soon you will be digitally surrounded by similar content, making it feel far and away the likeliest cause of any number of vague symptoms you might yourself be experiencing.

Long-Term Outcomes

Change in Health

When are your interventions likely to influence your patients' health understanding? We all try to make sense of changes in our health, and we tend to link them to events that preceded them. As in the example above, a patient may quickly come to believe that antibiotics cure sore throats if the clinician prescribes them with little explanation. In chronic illness, the possibility of recurrent consultations may build up helpful (or sometimes unhelpful) health beliefs. Ultimately, because we do not consult with most of our patients that often, we probably only play a small role in influencing our patients' health behaviour. The internet, social media, newspapers, family, and friends play a much larger role. The chance to influence their understanding will not arise very often, and we need to make the most of every opportunity that we have.

Medicalisation

This term describes the medical tendency to organise vague symptoms into categories, to label these categories, and produce a disease that can then be approached in the traditional medical manner. This tendency is particularly obvious in the medical handling of everyday emotional trauma; unhappiness is a human condition, whereas depression is a disease that can be treated pharmacologically and psychotherapeutically.

Labelling people creates illness. People who are found to have mild hypertension and who are told this fact suddenly have more sickness absence, have a higher incidence of impotence, cut down their participation in sport by over 50%, have double the incidence of panic attacks, and view themselves differently. This is before any possible drug side effects are manifested. Think about this for a moment. This means that all diagnoses have costs. To suddenly turn a person into a "hypertensive" is not a neutral event. Such a patient's perception of himself or herself has been altered quite markedly for the worse. Therefore, you must be quite certain that your diagnosis and subsequent intervention are going to outweigh the harm done.

There is also the medicalisation of daily living, where we see a society disinclined to manage simple, normal illness without consulting a professional, and lacking the medical knowledge that came from growing up in households with several generations of the same family, where shared experiences and wisdom provided the basis for a better understanding of health norms than most people have today.

If we as clinicians subscribe either consciously or unconsciously to this widespread tendency, it will affect both the way in which we consult and the outcomes of those consultations.

References

Cohen D. *Bad Influence: How the Internet Hijacked Our Health.* Oneworld Publications Ltd; 2026.

Kahneman D. *Thinking, Fast and Slow.* New York: Farrar, Straus and Giroux; 2011.

Little P. Observational study of effect of patient centredness and positive approach on outcomes of general practice consultations. *BMJ.* 2001;323:908.

Neighbour R. *The Inner Consultation.* 2nd ed. Oxford: Radcliffe Publishing; 2005.

Pereira Gray DJ. Continuity of care with doctors – A matter of life and death? A systematic review of continuity of care and mortality. *BMJ Open.* 2018;8:e021161.

CHAPTER

6

Different Methods of Consulting

The future is today.

William Osler, 1913

- Medicine takes place in a wide variety of clinical contexts.
- Technology is changing this landscape rapidly.
- Triage has become ubiquitous and differs from consulting.
- Whether triaging or consulting, do not lose sight of the central tenets of good communication – reaching a shared understanding and decision.
- Remember the therapeutic value of good communication.

The explosion in digital technology over recent years – coupled with shifts in patient behaviour and expectations, together with workload pressures in an increasingly busy NHS – has led to a rapid growth in alternatives to the traditional face-to-face consultation. Patients and clinicians can now communicate on the phone or by video call, via text or email or online form, sometimes with additional information such as photographs (we will bundle all these alternative methods under the umbrella term "remote contact"). Increasingly, technology in the form of algorithms and artificial intelligence is being interposed between the human beings involved. This rapidly evolving landscape can be bewildering to both patients and clinicians. Even where people feel confident and comfortable with the convenience

DOI: 10.1201/9781003652137-6

and productivity such innovations appear to offer, there may be pitfalls of which they are unaware.

To navigate this territory safely and effectively, there are three simple principles clinicians should keep in mind. One is the difference between triage and consultation. The second is the quality of communication inherent in the different methods of contact and how well this is suited to the matter in hand. The third is the importance of safety netting. The skills we have discussed over the previous chapters remain fundamentally important to all three principles.

Triage Versus Consultation

Generally, when a patient contacts the health service, they are seeking a consultation – they have a problem, and they have decided they need help in understanding and/or doing something about it. Patients are never seeking triage. The patient's agenda is a consultation.

Triage is something the health service does to patients in order to use its limited resources most effectively. Broadly speaking, it is a process that decides the timing, type, and location of a consultation, and what kind of professional is most appropriate to conduct it … or indeed whether a consultation is necessary at all. Triage is a health service agenda.

Over the past decade, triage has become virtually ubiquitous throughout primary care, both in and out of hours. Its advent has only become possible because of the array of remote contact methods now available. Health service resources have always been limited, and until recently they tended to be allocated by essentially arbitrary means: whether a patient could get through on the phone; when or whether any appointments were available if they did; how convincing they were when trying to persuade a receptionist to book them into one, etc. The aim of triage is to allocate these limited resources more rationally and along more clinically appropriate lines.

Triage works when it coincides with a shared understanding (even then, though, some patients will perceive it as one more barrier to surmount in their quest to achieve a consultation). Consider the following example. A 25-year-old swimming instructor is annoyed to have another bout of otitis externa, and experience tells her an ear spray will get rid of it. Taking time off work would involve cancelling classes, and she can't have her phone on her in the pool. The clinician reading her online e-consult is happy that her symptoms are typical – the algorithm working in the background has prompted for symptoms that might be concerning – and as well as sending a prescription electronically, the GP can text her safety-netting advice. Direct, real-time communication hasn't been necessary: the situation has been dealt with "asynchronously".

Such asynchronous shared understandings do occur, but they are far from the norm. Suppose instead the same instructor is worried about how often she gets ear infections. Her mother went deaf in her fifties: might her recurrent problems result in the same? Is there anything she can do to prevent the bouts, or should she look to change her career? Her Google research suggests multiple "ear infections" can lead to scarring of the ear drum: she's decided it's worth taking time off to have a doctor examine her and discuss the situation. She asks for a face-to-face review. The triaging GP is stressed by the numbers of e-consults piling up and the scarcity of appointments. She is faintly irritated that someone with classic otitis externa is bothering the service rather than going to a pharmacy. She skim-reads the free-text comments about deafness, pings off a prescription for Otomize, messages the patient to say any hearing loss will resolve once the infection clears and moves on to the next in the triage queue. The patient, dissatisfied, turns up later that evening in the ED, hoping that there she might actually get to see a human being to address her concerns. The casualty officer, stressed by the numbers stacking up in minors, is faintly irritated that someone with simple otitis externa should be bothering the service.

One reason this contact broke down is that the GP failed to appreciate the distinction between triage and consultation. In the first example, there was a shared understanding of the problem and what to do about it, and the triage outcome (health service agenda) mapped seamlessly onto the consultation outcome (patient's agenda). In the second case, the triage outcome was identical, but it failed to map onto a satisfactory consultation outcome. The main reason this happened was due to a narrow focus on the biomedical, which happens all too often with triage. Otitis externa is usually a trivial condition, and the algorithm had screened out concerning features, so it didn't appear to warrant a consultation. What the doctor failed to do was address the patient's ICE, thinking only of the biomedical aspects of the presentation.

As we have seen earlier in this book, consultations of any sort – even "gold standard" face-to-face consultations – that fail to address ICE generally don't end well. Except in the most urgent presentations, or straightforwardly transactional encounters, a sole focus on the biomedical is unlikely to result in a satisfactory outcome. *ICE is as important to triage as it is to consultation.* Both triage and consultation should, if possible, result in a shared understanding and decision about what to do.

It is worth touching on the fundamental difference between triage and consultation. A triage encounter isn't usually trying to arrive at a diagnosis and management; it is principally about deciding how and where and how quickly that process should take place. As such, the information gathered will often be briefer and more focused. The same symptom – abdominal pain, for example – might warrant an urgent face-to-face review or a routine appointment with the patient's usual GP, depending on whether it has come on that day or it is something the patient has been experiencing for the past year. But addressing the patient's ICE in the triage process is just as important as putting the presenting symptoms into biomedical context. That year-long history of abdominal pain might seem to warrant a routine review some weeks hence to the triaging clinician, but to a patient issued with a final warning over sickness absence from work, it could feel a great deal more pressing.

Sometimes, an encounter that starts as a triage morphs into a consultation when it becomes evident that the problem could be fully addressed at that point. It is very important that the clinician recognises when this is the case because more detail is likely to be required, sufficient to enable a safe diagnosis, differential, and shared management plan. It is hopefully obvious that this can't usually be done either without a correspondingly good understanding of the patient's ICE.

Quality of Communication

To achieve shared understanding in either triage or remote consultation, it's important to consider the quality of communication and to ask: is this appropriate to address the matter in hand? Let's consider the quality of communication in various scenarios.

Face to Face

The "gold standard". As we have seen, this affords both clinician and patient the full spectrum of human communication, verbal and non-verbal – and remember, the majority of interpersonal communication is non-verbal, the subtleties of eye contact, body posture, movement, all conveying much without words being spoken. Additionally, the patient is available for physical examination, another way in which their body can convey important information to the clinician.

Communication in a face-to-face consultation is "synchronous", happening in real time, which allows both clinician and patient to calibrate and adjust, to clarify and expand, according to how the consultation is unfolding – and ultimately to try to negotiate a shared understanding.

The main drawbacks to face-to-face encounters are inconvenience to the patient, who will usually have to arrange a specific time and then travel to attend, and potentially capacity issues for the health service. However, while it is often assumed that face-to-face appointments are the most time-inefficient, this is almost certainly not the case. For example, within seconds of seeing an ill child, or an adult with abdominal pain, most experienced clinicians can tell whether there is likely to be cause for concern, something that could take many minutes of information-gathering via a remote process.

Face to face is essentially inappropriate as a triage tool. Once a patient is in front of a clinician, a consultation is occurring and should be dealt with as such.

When comparing the various methods of remote contact with this "gold standard", there are two key factors to bear in mind: synchronicity and depth of communication.

Telephone

Telephone contact offers potential convenience to patients, especially with the near ubiquity of the mobile phone. There is no need to take time off work, arrange for someone to look after the children, or get in the car in order to seek medical care. The convenience aspect is tempered by unpredictability. When you're sitting in a surgery waiting room, all you're doing is expecting to be called through to a private room where you will be able to talk uninterrupted and in confidence. A phone call from a clinician, however, can come at an inconvenient time – in the middle of a lunch date, or while on the loo – which might affect the quality of a patient's communication through distraction or inhibition. Or frustratingly, the clinician's call might happen during the few short minutes when you were unable to answer – dealing with a child's temper tantrum, perhaps – and that might mean going to the back of the queue again. Even when connected, poor signal quality can hamper effective communication in either direction, as can the sense that many of us have that phone calls should be as brief as possible so that participants can get on with their day.

Telephony also deprives us of a large part of non-verbal communication, so both clinician and patient can miss important cues and nuances. Clinicians need to remain constantly alert to this and be sure it is not impairing their assessment. Additionally, we are "blind" to the environment the patient is in (who else might be in the room?) which can introduce a further layer of complexity. Some aspects of non-verbal communication are preserved, such as speech rate and tone, hesitations and pauses, repeated points. By paying close attention to the way things are said (and not said), clinicians can still gain valuable insights into what might be going on beneath the words – this is when active listening (as discussed in Chapter 4) can be so helpful in ensuring that we really are discovering the patient's agenda and reaching a shared understanding. The corollary is that patients, too, have lost much non-verbal communication – misunderstandings are more likely, so clinicians need to be particularly careful that their words aren't susceptible to being misconstrued ("I really don't think this is anything serious" could come across as dismissive on the phone, but delivered with eye contact, and a reassuring smile or touch, might be highly therapeutic).

The telephone was the first remote method to be widely used – it has been established as part of the workload mix in most general practices for decades, and some surgeries were already using the phone to triage all initial contacts prior to Covid. The exigencies of the pandemic turned "total triage" into the default position in NHS primary care for a couple of years, mainly using the phone, and very few practices have fully reverted to the way they used to work now that the pandemic has subsided, especially with the NHS GP contract changes stipulating the requirement for all patient contacts during core hours to be assessed on the day.

Telephone contact (once clinician and patient have managed to connect) has the advantage, like face to face, of being synchronous. In our second swimming instructor scenario, a phone call would have given the GP the opportunity to explore the patient's ICE properly. It might have remained as a triage call; the clinician could have prescribed ear spray for the immediate infection and arranged a routine face-to-face appointment to examine, discuss the family history further, and address her concerns for the longer term. Or it could have ended up as a telephone consultation, the patient being reassured that hearing loss from otitis externa is highly unlikely, some context being arrived at for her mother's history, and a shared decision being reached to trial methods of preventing water ingress into the ears as a next step.

Video Call

Much the same considerations apply to video consultations as telephone calls. The key difference is the restoration of some of the visual aspects of non-verbal communication, and a limited ability to examine some features such as rashes or skin lesions. The encounters are again synchronous, with the advantages this brings of being able to respond to the evolving picture and to negotiate shared understanding.

Interestingly, current experience suggests patients much prefer telephone over video contacts. Whether this is because a video call is a degree more intimate or intrusive – making patients feel they need to be smartly turned out, with no washing-up piled on the side in the kitchen – is unclear. Even a generation that has grown up with FaceTime, Skype, Zoom, and Teams may feel that video calls are most appropriate either for informal encounters (family, friends) or formal ones (interviews and work meetings), and medical consultations are perceived as falling somewhere awkwardly in between.

Where a video call offers some ability to examine the patient, it is important to be mindful how limited the quality of the "communication" their body can impart is. A rash that is typical for shingles might be diagnosable; a child seen haring round the living room behind their worried parent might be reassuring. But in most scenarios where examination is indicated, a face-to-face consultation should result. Subtle signs on abdominal palpation, positive neurology, or unexpected findings on chest auscultation are the stuff of medicine, and it would be an unwise clinician who fails to put themselves in a position to detect them.

To a limited extent, still images sent via text can aid remote assessment in the same way as a video call. These are most likely to be helpful with some rashes and skin lesions. But always ask yourself: is the quality of visual information appropriate? Out-of-focus photos, or lesions that need dermatoscopic evaluation, should be assessed in person.

Online Forms (e-Consult et al.)

An increasingly employed method of contact with primary care is via online tools such as e-Consult. The advantage for patients is they can (in theory) readily make contact with the practice without having to hold interminably on the phone. But here we are entering a different realm of communication that is both asynchronous and devoid of non-verbal dimensions.

The early simple proformas have been superseded by platforms with algorithms running in the background. These products prompt patients for biomedically relevant information: Is there fever with the rash? Is there vomiting with the abdominal pain? And so on. They also screen for "red flag" comments and divert patients automatically – for example, sending patients with chest pain into the emergency services at the point of first contact, rather than building in potential time delays in waiting for a clinician to be able to respond. This is very much a double-edged sword. All algorithms are risk averse, so along with the occasional STEMI or PE, they will overreact to symptoms that human clinicians would readily recognise as medically non-serious. This has adverse consequences for those patients whose problems ought to have been properly managed in primary care and has significant knock-on effects on pressure and costs elsewhere in the system (and when the patient with the PE gets to ED, their care may be delayed because of the backlog of costochondritis and panic attack cases).

Leaving aside the problem of these automatically diverted contacts, the background algorithms are trained on biomedical scenarios and their output is intended to provide clinicians with the relevant information to put the presenting symptom(s) into *biomedical context*. But remember these important things we learned earlier: patients don't contact the health service with a symptom, they do so with *ideas*, *concerns*, and *expectations* about that symptom; patients are never seeking triage, they are seeking a consultation; and ICE is as important to triage as it is to a consultation.

Online tools do prompt patients to enter any concerns they may have (the algorithms can't and don't factor these into their assessments; they are purely for human clinicians to consider). But how useful is this? Just as in traditional consultations, not all patients can or will state some or all of their ICE on an e-Consult form, always assuming they are even consciously aware of them (remember the concepts of *layering* and *reticence*, and the role of the subconscious that we met in Chapter 4). The strictly text-based nature of this communication means it is devoid of the cues that should lead an actively listening clinician to probe, explore, contextualise, and negotiate, and its asynchronicity is a profound barrier to doing so. This plays into exactly the problem we described earlier: ICE as a perfunctory box to be ticked and moved on from.

Online platforms clearly have a role as triage tools, though as we've seen from our swimming instructor they can lead to dysfunctional decisions due to their biomedical focus and the limitations they impose on a proper evaluation and incorporation of a patient's ICE. What is true for triage is an order of magnitude greater when considering their use for e-consultation. Remember the ultimate goal of a consultation: to arrive at a *shared understanding and shared management plan*. Sometimes every piece of information necessary for this is there, but often it is not. Clinicians should be constantly asking themselves: Has this online encounter become a consultation and, if so, have my patient and I come to a shared understanding of the problem and what to do about it? If the answers are yes and no respectively, then a different mode of consultation is required.

Text and Email

Platforms like AccuRx, which burst onto the scene during the Covid pandemic, have made texting a routine part of modern general practice. Most online tools have the capability to text or email patients directly from the platform. It can be a very useful way of dealing with simple problems or sending links to information for patients.

This can appeal to busy clinicians because of its apparent time efficiency. Maybe that ultrasound report came back with nothing abnormal on it: ping off a quick text with the good news. Sometimes this will suffice. But the very feature that can make it feel attractive to harried clinicians – you're not going to get tangled up with the patient asking lots of questions – is the reason it can fail. Unless the clinician authorises it, patients cannot respond by texting back: this is asynchronous and one-way communication. Be very sure this is appropriate in any instance in which it's employed. A good rule of thumb: never communicate a new diagnosis or abnormal test results by text or email – it's a rare patient who won't want to ask things or have a discussion.

Where the clinician authorises a patient to respond, this does introduce an element of synchronicity, albeit a clunky and episodic one. If you find yourself texting back and forth more than once or twice, it's telling you to arrange a synchronous form of contact. Texting has the same drawbacks as the online tools, in that all aspects of non-verbal communication are lost. The ability to enter free text removes any constraints that an online tool might impose, but the flipside is that there is nothing algorithmic guiding comprehensive and structured input.

Email is less frequently used but should be considered analogous to text. And in both cases, patients changing numbers or email addresses without updating their records is a potential problem.

A Word About AI

The dizzying advances in artificial intelligence (AI) in recent years are certain to transform many aspects of medicine. AI is particularly strong on pattern discernment in large data sets, and it is already assuming a place in fields such as radiology, histopathology, and population health analytics.

Its application to triage and consulting is a more nuanced beast. It remains largely biomedical in focus, and all experienced clinicians know how psychosocially complex most of our work is. Fed distilled biomedical information, AI can be impressive at differential diagnosis generation. The key point, though, is being "fed distilled biomedical information". AI is nowhere near able to translate the raw material our patients routinely impart. And the twin issues of safety and liability mean that it frequently overreacts, creating greater system expense and patient inconvenience. The first algorithmic application to healthcare in the United Kingdom was NHS Pathways, the software used by NHS 111 non-clinical call handlers. This continues to designate around ten times more patients as urgent and emergency cases than an experienced GP would do. The large language models (LLMs) such as ChatGPT that have soared in popularity over the past few years create deceptively anthropomorphic output, making it appear that they are able to reason. For all this appearance of sentience, however, they are at heart no more than extremely powerful probabilistic prediction machines. Recent research has shown that their diagnostic precision degrades markedly when trying to interpret unrefined real-world information from human patients (Bean et al., 2026), or when confronted by unfamiliar scenarios that don't match patterns in their training data (Bedi et al., 2025). If you consider how vanishingly rarely patients present with "textbook cases" in day-to-day practice, you can see the pitfalls in relying on LLMs for decisions of any consequence.

Beyond its limitations as a diagnostic tool, though, can AI replicate what we have demonstrated throughout this book: the therapeutic nature of good communication, the complexities and nuances of the interaction between clinician and patient, and the prime importance of shared understanding? Adam Phillips and Simon Rudland describe what they term "Post-Turing Clinical Relationships" (2026) – an increasingly common phenomenon in which people form ongoing dialogues with an LLM over their health issues, influencing how they interpret symptoms, modulate their degree of anxiety, and make decisions over whether and when to seek clinical care. There can be positive aspects: one of us has recent experience of a young female patient with torrid diarrhoea-predominant IBS who, once diagnosed in medical consultation, found both helpful validation and useful dietary manipulations through subsequent engagement with ChatGPT. But there are pitfalls. LLMs are engineered to produce output aligned to the prompts that users input – the precise reason they appear so empathic, collaborative, and "on your side". There are already several tragic documented examples of LLMs encouraging and facilitating suicide in individuals with depression, and Ro Woon Lee and colleagues (2025) have shown how easily LLMs can be induced to offer inappropriate or dangerous medical advice – including recommending thalidomide in pregnancy. We stated earlier in this book that an entirely patient-focused clinician is probably a dangerous creature. It seems to us that LLMs, by their design, veer very much in that direction. Chris Whitty, England's chief medical officer, has expressed concern that GPs are having to spend significant consultation time "undoing" incorrect information that LLMs have confidently given patients. While we applaud Whitty for raising the issue, contemporary clinicians don't need to be unduly fazed or alarmed by this novel phenomenon. As we have shown, elicitation and exploration of patients' ICE has long been fundamental to effective consultations, and post-Turing clinical relationships are just a new variation on the way in which patients' ICE are formed.

It is that connection between clinician and patient trying to share understanding and with a common goal that is so vital. The clinician's objectivity, born of training, experience, and professional judgement, is every bit as important to that process as their empathic understanding of patient perspectives. Human clinicians do not need to fear for their jobs any time soon.

Safety Netting

Safety nets are vital and improve the overall safety of any encounter, be it triage or consultation, face to face or remote. But safety netting is arguably of prime importance with remote contacts, given the varied quality of the communication that each method entails.

Too often clinicians forget the essence of good communication when establishing a safety net. They will reel off extensive lists of things that might just happen, presumably because they mistake the net as being for clinician rather than patient safety – "I've mentioned every possible contingency anyone could think of, so I'm medicolegally secure should things not work out as expected". The literature abounds with studies illustrating that patients remember very little of the information or advice they're given in a consultation – much of what is said in supposedly comprehensive safety netting will sail straight over the patient's head and is completely worthless, both practically and medicolegally.

Good safety netting involves continued excellent communication. If it's possible to make general statements, these are better than long lists. So, in the case of a patient five days into a viral URTI, try saying: "I don't expect you to develop any new symptoms, or to feel worse from here, so if you do, you should contact us for further advice". If there are specific important points to watch for, we'd suggest keeping them to, at most, three: "I don't expect your child to develop a rash, or to start vomiting, or to become unusually drowsy". If it's important to get additional things across, repeat and chunk: "So rash, vomiting, and unusual drowsiness are three symptoms to watch for. In addition, it's important they stay hydrated. Keep an eye on the amount they're peeing. You should see at least two wet nappies a day".

Having pared the safety net down to the most crucial details, ask the patient or carer to repeat it back to you. "It's important to check you've got all that. Would you mind telling me what you're going to watch out for?" They might come back with a perfect rendition, but more often they will skip certain points, which you can then repeat and reinforce.

Finally, remember that, just as with every other aspect of the consultation, the goal is a shared understanding and decision, so check you've achieved this. Avoid asking closed questions that entail potential disagreement or conflict. "Does that seem an OK plan?" might sound friendly, but if the patient has any misgivings, they're going to have to steel themselves to tell the clinician, "no, it doesn't". Enquire instead how the patient or carer feels. "I've been through quite a lot with you. How confident are you about managing the situation? Do you have any misgivings?"

All these techniques will help ensure the robustness of a safety net.

Out-of-Hours Working

The out-of-hours (OOH) setting has some key differences to routine consulting. This cohort of patients has self-selected as those who cannot wait to be seen routinely, and there is a higher incidence of acute organic pathology as well as greater levels of anxiety and stress. Tools such as GP Connect are at last allowing OOH clinicians to view a summary of the primary care record, but even so, one is often dealing with sick or fearful patients with minimal additional information. This is inherently risky, as reflected by the enhanced premiums charged by the medical defence organisations for such work. Increasing demand has affected all areas of the health service in recent years, and the advent of NHS 111 has driven increased workload into OOH services. Patient volumes can be high, and a balance between speed and thoroughness can be difficult to strike. When there are few, if any, records to rely on, our history-taking and communication skills become even more important. We do not have that knowledge or experience of a patient to fall back on or to allow us to place the patient before us into context. It is inevitable that we practise more cautiously in these settings, but we must be wary not to be too cautious and expose patients to over-investigation and unnecessary treatments. Once again, good communication is key. Involve patients and relatives where you are able, remember to keep sharing and checking understanding, make a shared decision, and have a really sturdy safety net.

General Points to Consider

However you might be communicating with a patient, remember to introduce yourself clearly. Even a patient who knows you may not recognise you from voice alone on the phone. Text or email signatures should clearly state your details.

Just as in a face-to-face consultation, patients can be upset, rude, or aggressive during a telephone call (or any remote contact method). Some people feel the relative anonymity means they can be as rude as they like. Try to keep in mind that illness is frequently stressful and frightening, which can affect how people behave. Counter any antagonism by empathising with how they're feeling. Introduce a human element, reminding them that you are a real person, not just a voice or a text correspondent, and that you are trying to help. However, setting boundaries is important, and if poor behaviour continues, this is not acceptable. There is no room in modern-day medicine for abuse, and we should have a zero-tolerance attitude towards those who behave inappropriately.

Remote consulting is made safer when identifying those consultations in which it is *not* safe. Patients who cannot communicate for themselves are most at risk, including children, those whose carers phone on their behalf, or those in residential or nursing care homes. For some of these patients, remote consultations with a third party on their behalf can be entirely appropriate, but for many it will not be, and part of the skill is to know when a problem cannot be safely managed in this way. And remember, sometimes actually being able to eyeball the patient for a minute or two gives you more information than half an hour spent on the telephone, no matter how effective your communication skills. We feel this point is worth repeating.

Patients with mental health conditions may be especially short-changed by the lack of face-to-face contact with an empathic and listening fellow human being. Much of the mental state examination relies on visual and aural information, which is variously compromised by the different remote contact methods. This is not to say that it is impossible to be empathic and to listen via a video or telephone consultation, but we need to acknowledge that it is harder to do so effectively. That said, unpublished survey results by one of our GP registrars found that a majority of patients with mental health difficulties reported preferring phone consultation, perhaps because the aura of anonymity made it easier to speak openly about feelings and very personal issues.

The rise of remote contact methods may have an impact on the public's perception of the need to access healthcare. Having the convenience of a clinician just a tap away on your smartphone represents a far lower "barrier" to seeking care than having to arrange time out of normal life to attend surgery. Are we promoting a culture of over-reliance on medical advice and a lack of public understanding about the importance of their own role in being responsible for their health? Consider the potential for game-savvy patients to learn to play the various systems. These patients learn how to avoid continuity and consult with multiple clinicians (so-called doctor shopping). Internet forums for specified conditions are an increasingly used guide to such strategies; doctors, particularly GPs, are usually not well portrayed in such sites. We must be aware of this risk and protect patients from the well-known, substantial, and significant harms of over-medicalisation. While it is not yet clear what the impact of remote contacts on continuity of care is, the concern is that a lack of continuity will make for less effective medicine. Healthcare is again risking being reduced to a transaction, a simple exchange of information and the provision of treatment or tests, rather than the genuine sharing of understanding that we have demonstrated is so fundamentally important.

Conclusion

Remote methods of triage and consultation are here to stay, and they do carry some advantages for both patient and clinician. In order to navigate this landscape safely and effectively, remember these key points:

- Patients want consultations; triage is a health service agenda.
- ICE is important to both activities.
- Consider the synchronicity and depth of communication inherent in the different methods of contact, and ensure they match the needs of the presentation.
- Safety netting is vital, and if it is to be effective, it demands the same high standards of communication as every other aspect of patient–doctor interaction.

References

Bean AM et al. Reliability of LLMs as medical assistants for the general public: a randomized preregistered study. *Nat Med.* 2026. https://doi.org/10.1038/s41591-025-04074-y

Bedi S et al. Fidelity of Medical Reasoning in Large Language Models. *JAMA Netw Open* 2025;8(8):e2526021.

Lee RW et al. Vulnerability of Large Language Models to Pompt Injection When Providing Medical Advice. *JAMA Netw Open* 2025;8(12):e2549963.

Osler W. *A Way of lLife.* New Haven, CT: Yale University Press; 1913. p. 19.

Phillips A and Rudland S. *BJGP life*; 2026. https://bjgplife.com/post-turing-clinical-relationships-how-ai-is-reshaping-patient-behaviour-before-the-consultation/

CHAPTER 7

Complex Scenarios

What is spoken of as a clinical picture is not just a photograph of a sick man in bed; it is an impressionistic painting ... surrounded by his home, his work, his relations, his joys, sorrows, hopes, and fears.

Francis Peabody

- Some consultations require much more effort than others.
- The concept of different agendas can be an important aid to navigating complexity.
- No matter how challenging, focus on the key outcomes that you want to achieve.
- Keep your consultation style fluid and adjust it to suit the patient/situation in front of you.

So far in this book we have explored the importance of tailoring your communication to the patient and clinical situation, and the need to explore their understanding and perspectives. In this chapter we will delve further into some more complex, specific scenarios where the clinician needs to consider additional factors.

DOI: 10.1201/9781003652137-7

Children and Their Parents/Carers

For obvious reasons, almost all children will be brought to a consultation by an adult carer – most usually a parent or parents but sometimes other caregivers, relatives, or friends. Get into the habit of recording who is present at each consultation; occasionally this can be important retrospective information.

It is generally a mistake – or at the very least, a missed opportunity – to focus exclusively on the adults' contribution. Clearly the amount a young patient can articulate and explain will vary considerably with age – there's no useful history to be obtained from a toddler – with the individual child's character and confidence, and with the nature of the presenting complaint (mental health, behavioural, dietary, or neurodiversity concerns usually come from parents). Nevertheless, except in the case of the very young, it is well worth giving your child patient the opportunity to play an active role in the consultation – children as young as three are capable of quite complex thought and communication, and patients as young as eight or ten years sometimes competently conduct proceedings with minimal input from their accompanying adult.

Your approach has to be age-appropriate and to be calibrated in real time according to how things unfold, but a good starting point in most circumstances is to introduce yourself to your child patient, check what they like to be called, and ask who they've brought along with them (you'll usually be met with a sudden smile and the news that the grown-up sitting next to them is "Mummy!" or "Daddy!"). You can then ask how you can help and sit back and see how things develop. Sometimes the child will quickly defer to their parent, but you'll be surprised how often you'll get a good sense of the history from the patient themselves before their caregiver decides they need to chip in. Staying alert to body language cues from both parent and child should allow you to switch between them fluidly and appropriately. Almost all children relish being treated as a "grown-up", and generally, parents appreciate their offspring being given the opportunity to be involved in their own healthcare too.

That said, particularly for younger children, it will usually be the parent who has well-formed ICE that will need to be uncovered for the consultation to conclude successfully, so after gaining a good history, your focus will often shift to address parental perspectives. Be especially alert to non-verbal cues because parents may be reluctant to express certain ideas or concerns if they think it would upset their child. Always consider parental concerns carefully and respond to them collaboratively, even if on the face of it they seem unlikely: these are the people who know their child better than anyone. And don't neglect to elicit any ICE that the child may have themselves. Illness can be just as worrying for a young person as an adult – sometimes more so – and they will often have been researching symptoms online or fearing that something serious is going on.

Equally, when explaining your thoughts or outlining a proposed plan, address both child (other than the very youngest) and carer. Your language and concepts will need to be pitched at an appropriate level for your child patient, but most parents will readily translate what you're saying into "adult speak" and will let you know they're doing so through nods and eye contact. More complex information or safety netting may need to be expanded upon directly to the parent, and this is perfectly appropriate, but be aware that your child patient will be listening closely and may comprehend more than you'd imagine, so keep monitoring their body language to gauge their reaction. In certain circumstances – for example, where a child's presenting symptoms are reflecting their emotional response to circumstances within the family or school – it may be appropriate to arrange a separate conversation with their caregivers.

It is important to bear in mind that a child's and a parent's agendas may be very different, and that a parent's presence in the consultation can sometimes be inhibitory. By being mindful of the substance of the issue being presented, and alert to non-verbal cues, you should readily develop a sense of circumstances in which it might be important to talk to the child on their own. Engineering this can be delicate – while you don't want to force a child into a solo conversation if they're not comfortable, there is no point asking them in front of the parent if they would like to speak to you alone. If their parent is an inhibitory presence, the child will be inhibited when answering your question! So, if you decide that one-to-one time is important to your assessment, request it directly of the parent and ask them to take a seat in the waiting room; it is rare that you will be refused (and that itself may be significant). Once alone with your child patient, you can check if they're comfortable and if necessary, explain your reasons before proceeding. Your opening approaches to the consultation will prove to have been very valuable in these circumstances, helping to gain the child's trust and confidence from the outset.

The frequency and nature of the problems with which a child is brought for consultation will often reflect the parent or caregiver's health beliefs and personality. Parents are usually hard-wired to be anxious about and protective of their offspring's health and will frequently be fearful of something serious underlying the presentation, or of it being missed by professionals. Be especially alert to this where the objective clinical picture is at odds with the degree of concern – it is vital to discover the parent's ICE in order to achieve a successful outcome. And always bear in mind that the child patient may be the symptom of parental ill-health – the repeated presentations with minor ailments indicating post-natal depression or anxiety, for example. Foster carers frequently have a low threshold for seeking professional assessment, and understanding the obligations and responsibilities they carry towards their foster child can provide important context.

Conflict between child and parent agendas sometimes arises because of differing views about medical treatment. All children aged 16–17 years are presumed competent to consent, and those under 16 may be able to, depending on their Gillick competence. Rather akin to mental capacity, Gillick competence is not a fixed entity, but depends on factors such as the child's intelligence, maturity, ability to understand information and options, and the gravity of the decision being taken. It is also, as with mental capacity, decision-specific, meaning that a child who is competent to make one decision may lack this capacity in another situation. This means an assessment of Gillick competence is vital in each scenario. The techniques for doing so are well covered in good Mental Capacity Act training, and are outside the scope of this chapter. Where disagreement over treatment between a child and their parents – for example, contraceptive provision – occurs, keep uppermost in mind your duty of confidentiality to your competent child patient. Listening carefully to all perspectives is important – parental concerns are every bit as valid as teenage self-determination and may yield vital considerations such as the age of the sexual partner. Through non-judgemental and respectful communication, it may be possible to help negotiate a resolution to the conflict, but ultimately in the case of a competent child one's duty is primarily to them. Good documentation in these scenarios is vital; these decisions can be tricky and nuanced, and being able to justify why you have made them is occasionally necessary.

Consultations with More Than One Person Present

This is a challenging area of communication and has existed since the invention of medicine. Patients who attend with other family or friends are perhaps the most frequent example (other than the aforementioned children). Again, always note who is present for each consultation.

The dynamics of communication are very different when a third party or more parties participate, but the central aim remains to achieve a shared understanding based on your and their medical knowledge; it is just harder.

First, check consent. Just because the spouse has followed the patient into the room does not mean the patient wants them there or feels able to talk freely with them present. Be alert to the possibility of coercive, controlling behaviour or domestic or honour-based violence – the perpetrator will often accompany the victim to ensure their silence. This can be challenging to manage and, as alluded to in the last chapter, can be even more so in remote consultations.

Start by thinking of agendas, but whose? There is that of the "patient" (and it may not always be entirely clear who that is, or how many there are), the other party or parties, and of course the clinician's. Take the example of the wife bringing her reluctant 66-year-old husband to see you, concerned about his deteriorating memory. He doesn't perceive there to be a problem and declares bitterly that she is just "fussing". She is palpably frustrated by his comment, explaining that he keeps forgetting to do things, and is forever repeating the same old stories over and over again. Is this early dementia or one of a myriad of other possibilities – including, perhaps, a long-married couple adjusting to post-retirement life? Is he genuinely unconcerned, or might he be fearful and in denial as to what is happening? How is he going to react if you suggest a memory assessment and further investigations? She may be frightened about what his apparent memory difficulties mean for both their futures, convinced that treatment might improve things, and perhaps her anxiety is compounding the situation between them. Your agenda might be affected by feeling daunted at the breadth of the biopsychosocial differentials, a dislike of conflict, the challenge of negotiating a shared approach, and your heart might be sinking at how much time this scenario could take to disentangle amid all the other work you have to do that day. There is no prescriptive template for navigating these situations, but there are some good rules of thumb that should help achieve a good outcome.

Good and Bad Communication Strategies with More than One Person Present

Good

- Keeping confidentiality issues uppermost in your mind.
- Greeting each individual in such a way as to encourage their participation.
- Ensuring that each person feels their perspectives are heard.

- Being on the lookout for and acknowledging the emotions expressed (positive and negative).
- Trying to control monopolisation and persistent interruptions.
- Splitting complex scenarios where possible into multiple consultations to create time and opportunity to develop your understanding fully.
- Remembering that you may have more than one "patient" in front of you.
- Recognising that you will have your own agenda, and guarding against it affecting the consultation.

Not So Good

- Assuming that the person whose appointment it is, is the only "patient".
- Stopping the story too soon.
- Letting one individual regularly speak for another.
- Taking sides.
- Offering advice without fully exploring the problem.
- Leaving the computer screen notes of one patient available for another to view.
- Allowing negative aspects of your own agenda to influence your handling of the consultation.

Consulting Through an Interpreter

Interpretation is a necessity whenever a patient's English is not sufficient for effective communication. This is not an area of particular expertise for us, and there are publications dedicated solely to this, but a few of the more important points are covered here.

First, interpreted consultations take longer, so make sure you have additional time allocated. Using a professional interpreting service such as Language Line will *at least* double the appointment length because the interpreter will be translating every question and answer in each direction. Consultations where a family member interprets may feel preferable because they will usually be swifter (the patient and family member will usually have been developing their understanding of the problem prior to attending and rather than translating, the family member might try to speak for the patient) but these are generally undesirable for the reasons we will come to.

Whoever is interpreting, you must be aware that your patient may omit important parts of the history because of embarrassment or worries about confidentiality. Being overtly clear to patients about their confidentiality when consulting with a professional interpreter can help to diffuse this. In circumstances where a family member is interpreting, you self-evidently cannot make any comment about confidentiality and the risks are even higher: there are many things that an older parent, for example, will not want to disclose in front of their adult child.

When talking to a patient through an interpreter, remember to keep looking at the patient. It may be harder to pick up on the verbal cues, but the visual ones are still there. Make sure the patient understands that you are genuinely interested in them, not the interpreter, and that you are trying to understand them. Focus on using open questions, as it can be much easier to quickly move on to closed questions which are simpler for the translator. Sometimes this is needed, but it is at the expense of giving the patient the opportunity to tell you what they are worried about. This is not easy, and may well take a lot of time, but your consultation will be more effective for it.

If a family member is doing the interpreting, then there is an extra layer of complexity. Professional medical interpreters will tell you what the patient has said; family members are likely to paraphrase or tell you their own interpretation or perspective, which dilutes the patient's meaning. This is normally done with the best of intentions, but it can be done in a controlling or, worse, malicious way; for example, the domestic violence victim whose abusive partner is the interpreter. Be aware of and look out for these risks and, where possible, use a professional interpreter.

AI now offers potential interpretation solutions. Applications like Google Translate can be useful for identifying specific words or phrases, but typing during a consultation will generally slow things to a snail's pace. Speech-to-text technology is far wieldier and there are impressive apps that can translate spoken input in one language into both written and verbal output in another, and vice versa. A caution with all such applications: none are designed or approved as "medical grade" and can consequently generate potentially important miscommunication. One of us conducted consultations with a 67-year-old Polish patient via his speech-to-text app and at one point learned that he was having problems with his dad. This initially seemed unsurprising: his father may well have been a nonagenarian. Trying to establish the nature of the difficulties – was it dementia, or advanced frailty – resulted in increasingly puzzling exchanges, until eventually the penny dropped. "Dad" was an unfortunate mistranslation of a Polish euphemism for the male member. Thereafter, progress was made with managing the prostate problems that were making it increasingly difficult to pee.

With all of these variables, consulting across languages can be rather like consulting while wearing a motorcycle helmet with a dirty visor. Familiar signals may not mean the same thing, eye contact may be abhorred, a nod may not indicate acceptance, and so on, so your only resort is to keep checking your patient's understanding as best you can.

Breaking Bad News

This is one of the most difficult aspects of medical practice. Start by returning to the concept of agendas and focus for a moment on your own. Many clinicians find breaking bad news a daunting prospect, and the reasons are usually emotional. Causing distress in another person causes distress in us. Therefore, many of us do not perform very well in this crucial area of medical communication. We would ideally like not to have to do it, and if we do find ourselves having to do it, we can all too easily deploy strategies that protect us emotionally, but which do not serve our patient well.

Common methods of "just not doing this" include avoiding the patient, never seeing them alone, or always being in a hurry. Trainees in hospital are exposed to this dilemma all the time. Virtually every encounter with an acutely unwell patient involves breaking bad news in some form, and many prefer to gloss over it, dress it up, or simply sidestep the issue entirely. This is largely out of fear and lack of experience. There is also a vague feeling that "important" jobs such as this could be done better by someone more senior or that perhaps they are someone else's job. It is important to be alert to your own feelings, and if you recognise you are avoiding a bad news scenario, do something about it. If you feel you lack the knowledge to enter into the discussion, seek advice and support from a colleague and rehearse the situation, or do some background revision about the specific condition so that you feel better prepared.

Common self-protective strategies include unwarranted optimism, for example implying that a cure is possible, or that the patient is in "good hands, and we'll soon get you back on your feet" when you know that is not ultimately going to be the case. A corollary is brutal bluntness, where a clinician will unload the news in one stark go, often falling back on overly technical language (to obscure true meaning), under the justification that they are being "honest". Another frequent approach is to control the consultation so as to avoid uncomfortable issues. Studies have shown that clinicians frequently use closed questions and seldom give the patients space to initiate any discussion when breaking bad news.

Useful Strategies to Help You Break Bad News to Patients

Remember that for the patient this is a momentous occasion. People recall the how, where, and when very clearly, and you – as the clinician – are wielding immense power. Make sure you are unhurried and have a good amount of time. Arrange the appointment at the end of a surgery; or if on the ward, come back after the round. Consider offering to record the consultation. This technique is now being used with increasing frequency in oncology departments (less so in general practice, but perhaps that will change). The evidence suggests that the patients and their relatives listen to the recordings on several occasions (Pitkethly et al., 2008).

Generally, starting by asking what the patient knows about the situation will give you a good idea of where they are, both information-wise and psychologically. You can then build on that gently and as appropriate. Be especially sensitive: abrupt and brutal honesty, associated with authoritarian patient control, has no place in modern medicine. Choose your language with care. Whatever the words "cancer", "tumour", "growth", "metastases", "malignant", etc., mean to you, it is virtually certain that they do not mean the same thing to your patient. Check their understanding frequently, and remember that some people, cultures, and societies have taboos relating to words like cancer. Be careful.

Give your patient space to take it in. Pause, touch, empathise, commiserate, and above all don't be afraid to use silence. Allow your patient time to think of questions, and then you must answer them and assure them of ongoing support. Be prepared to spread the explanations over several consultations; it can help to ask the patient to write down questions as they come into their head and to bring them along to the next consultation. It is much better if bad news is given in the context of a continuing, supportive relationship.

Honesty is the only policy: never tell patients anything that you know is not true. This applies equally to situations where the diagnosis is not fully established. If a CT has come back looking ominous, for example, explain that you're concerned about cancer and that further tests are needed, but keep within the bounds of what is currently known. Do not, however, tell the patient more than they want to know. This implies the need for a skilful manoeuvre to find out how much information they can cope with. Try asking: "People vary a lot in how much they want to know about what's going on. Some want everything spelled out in detail, others are happy with broad brushstrokes. Where are you on that spectrum?"

Take great care with prognostications. *Never* give a specific time period – it will only come back to haunt you – but broad categories can be useful ("I think we're probably looking at a few weeks to a couple of months", "Depending on how you respond to treatment, this might be kept under control even for a year or two"). If your patient asks, "How long have I got?" they are probably already formulating an answer. You could say something like, "Well, I know you are poorly, but I think you have some time left. How does it look to you?" Their answer may help you to deepen the discussion.

Do not remove all hope. The condition may be terminal, but you can encourage the patient to look forward to a particular event, such as a birth or celebration of an anniversary, or they may be hoping for a period of remission or for a peaceful, pain-free death. Offer ongoing support wherever possible. Following up after giving bad news is especially important.

Remember the duty of confidentiality that is owed to your patient. This tends to go out of the window as soon as serious illness is suspected. Clinicians have become used to ushering spouses into darkened corners and whispering intimate details of their loved one's condition without a by-your-leave to the unfortunate sufferer. This has always been assumed to be for the patient's wellbeing. Almost all patients, however ill, want to know their diagnosis, and most of them want to know about the prognosis, treatment options, and side effects. Patients dislike unconditional disclosure of information without their consent; their own needs take priority over those of their family.

Make sure you give yourself some "housekeeping" time after the consultation, and consider debriefing with a colleague. This can be emotionally painful for you, too.

A Word About Denial

We all deal with devastating news in different ways. Many people cope by using varying degrees of denial. You will sometimes experience situations where you have what you consider to be a sensitive, honest chat with a patient, containing a great deal of information, and then at the next consultation the patient will appear to have absolutely no recollection of what was said.

It is not a good strategy to break down denial too brutally. It is there for a purpose. Respect for the individual should extend to their defence mechanisms. This does not mean that we ourselves have to be a party to the denial and start encouraging unrealistic expectations. We must still reply honestly to any questions. It also means that we must navigate patient cues carefully, such as "The consultant said it was just a little tumour. What a relief it isn't cancer!" A comment like that might represent denial, and you wouldn't want to crush it, but it can also be an oblique way for a patient to check that things really are as bad as they seem. If you collude and say something like, "Yes, that must be a relief", then you may build a false picture. Try reflecting back: "What did you understand the consultant to mean when they said 'tumour'?" If they want to know more, they will usually tell you what it meant to them but ask you if that is right or not. Take things in slow steps and with care.

Some patients decline to participate in shared decisions about end-of-life care. Typically, a bit of time spent exploring the patient's beliefs and expectations helps them move to a more realistic place where they can address the future pragmatically. Often, our patients are relieved by achieving this degree of acceptance and open participation in end-of-life decisions. But there will be occasions where it is apparent that ongoing denial is an important coping mechanism, and this must be respected. Keep this under sensitive review because it will often change over time.

Family denial or collusion is another problem more commonly encountered in general practice. This can lead to a tragic conspiracy of silence. The sufferer knows full well that their condition is terminal, but they cannot talk to their loved ones for fear of upsetting them. The loved ones, in turn, are so afraid of upsetting the sufferer in their last few weeks that nothing about the illness, about dying, about saying goodbye, etc., is discussed – to the detriment of all concerned. Collusion is always a two-way process. Here we think there is a place for sensitive intervention by the clinician to try to break this pernicious circle. We firmly believe that our responsibility is to the patient, and that any responsibility to the family is secondary. In the situation where a family pleads for keeping bad news from the patient, we should tell the relatives that we would not impose the truth, but that if the patient asks, we will not lie. Often, with experience and tact, we can persuade all parties to talk reasonably openly about the future and help the patient towards a better death, with a normal and not exaggerated grief to follow. This facilitation of family dynamics can be one of the more satisfying events in which we can become involved.

The Dying Patient and Bereavement

The care of a dying patient is a complex area where we need to utilise all of our communication skills effectively to gauge and provide the level of support that patients and their families need. The skills described around breaking bad news are needed throughout this particular clinical scenario as we try to inform, support, and counsel our dying patient. Overtly discussing their ideas, concerns, and expectations is vital. Unless we know what is important to that particular patient, it is difficult to provide comfort. Listening to patients and their families is a huge, central part of palliative care.

Advanced care planning is better understood by those outside the speciality of palliative care than it was a decade or two ago, including the benefits that most patients derive from being offered the opportunity to discuss what matters to them. Advanced care planning is commonly used in palliative care settings and is now also mainstream in general practice. Our hospital colleagues may have less experience, but even in the realms of the intensive care unit the need for advanced care planning is being recognised, as discussed by Jamie Gross in the *BMJ* (Gross et al., 2018).

Many patients and their families find that a frank, open discussion about what happens, and what to expect, when someone dies is very useful. Unless we ask patients what they want to know, we risk misinterpreting their silence. Clinicians have varying degrees of experience of looking after dying patients, but it will almost inevitably be greater than our patients' experience. In modern, especially Western, societies, death is much less visible than it was a century or so ago, and the general public does not usually have much experience of the changes that take place. The anorexia of advanced dementia or advanced cancer can be distressing to relatives, whereas clinicians recognise this as a sign of end-stage illness. Our understanding can provide comfort when communicated sensitively.

Looking after patients who have been bereaved can be very challenging. Grief can be raw, angry, emotional, and painful for those going through it, and painful to witness. Communication here is fundamental. We need to understand what has happened, the context of the loss, and the impact of the bereavement. Different people grieve in different ways, even within the same family, and those suffering a significant loss for the first time will often know little or nothing about the phases and duration of normal grief. Simply listening can be the most powerful, helpful tool, as can normalising their feelings and experiences, and offering the expectation of eventual resolution.

Angry Patients

This is another difficult emotional area, especially if the anger is directed towards you or one of your colleagues. Being ill can make people angry, so clinicians are going to encounter a lot more than their fair share of this emotion. Patients may be angry because we do not agree with them or will not do what they have demanded. Their anger may be directed at the system rather than the individual clinician, including excessive waiting times and delayed appointments, but we are the unfortunate recipients. Distress for another, often mixed with righteous indignation about perceived medical failings, sometimes results in very intense and unpleasant encounters. There may be concerns that what the patient feels has not been taken seriously, disappointment at the lack of therapeutic success, and simple misunderstandings (especially when the patient expects one treatment but receives another, and the clinician has failed to explain the rationale). Guilt felt by patients or relatives that, somehow, they should have come sooner or cared for the patient better is a common reason for anger being directed at clinicians. Anger is natural in grief and when adjusting to a serious diagnosis – the "why me?" effect. For most angry patients and relatives, anxiety or fear is often the trigger.

Strategies for Recognising and Dealing with Angry Patients

Consider the environment. If someone is sounding off in a public space like the waiting room, where other patients will be onlookers, offer to go somewhere private so you can talk and understand what's been happening. Taking people to a quieter area reduces their arousal and signifies that you are concentrating on them.

Anger may be overt, but sometimes it is there seething beneath the surface of a consultation. Use your own feelings to tell you how the patient is feeling. If you are feeling angry (which will often arise because you sense your competence or integrity being questioned), it is very likely that the patient is, too. Do not leave the anger unexplored. Remember that it is the patient/relative/carer who is angry, not you. This may be difficult, depending on your temperament, but try to cultivate the same kind of objective approach you would with other emotional states. Faced with a patient with tears brimming in their eyes, for example, we might reflect to them: "You look very upset. Can you tell me what's going on?" Try the same with anger.

Be patient – anger does not usually last for long. In communication terms, anger has a purpose – to gain the listener's (in this case the clinician's) complete attention. It is wise to let this happen. Allow them to vent, but within reason – a few patients will keep going for as long as you give them. Someone who is so angry they are ranting might need quite an assertive approach: "I really want to help sort this out, but I need you to tell me what exactly has been happening – can you talk me through it from the beginning?"

When you are listening, maintain non-threatening eye contact. Try not to raise your eyebrows, purse your lips or adopt an aggressive stance. When you speak, break off eye contact from time to time to demonstrate your wish to be conciliatory. An effective technique for dealing with angry people involves matching their communication style. The idea is that you can help to de-escalate the situation by matching them closely and then, once you are in control, shifting and bringing them with you. Try to subtly match their position (without obviously mimicking them which will probably annoy them further). If they are standing up and you are sitting down, there is an imbalance. You will feel more vulnerable, and they will feel more powerful. Stand up yourself and then perhaps if things are going well try sitting down and see if they follow suit. If not, stand up again. Try to match their demeanour. Obviously, avoid shouting yourself, but if they are talking loudly and you try to respond in a timid meek voice there is an imbalance. Raise your voice a bit until you are both on a level, then try to bring theirs down with you.

Once you have a good sense of the grievance(s), summarise the main points and then check them. Deal with the main issue first. Thank them for their response: "Thanks for being so honest/flagging the problem to me". Tempting as it is to jump in with defences and refutations, particularly when we are being criticised personally, it is much better to empathise and validate: "I can see how difficult that must have been for you" and "I am sure if I were in your position I would feel angry, too". It is surprising how effective this can be. Apologise sincerely (but do not accept the blame unless it really is your fault) – phrases like "I am so sorry to hear what's happened/what's been going on for you" can be helpful. Be diplomatic and show a genuine desire to resolve the issue. Always be professional, do not rise to the bait or become emotional. Do not get defensive or into an argument.

Try to offer solutions if appropriate. The reason for anger will dictate the way it is managed. Someone who is angry at a missed diagnosis will need time to vent, and an explanation as to the frailties and imperfections of medical diagnosis and treatment, an apology if warranted and then careful exploration of their understanding and next steps. Watch for the effects of your own guilt feelings. If something has gone wrong, or even if it hasn't (perhaps you saw a child with non-specific abdominal pain that the following day had evolved into recognisable appendicitis), feelings of guilt can make us reluctant to address the issue. But it is important to override these – you will often be met with understanding, and an improved relationship can result. Someone who is angrily demanding a prescription for methadone, however, will need a different approach involving careful negotiation and an understanding that a shared decision may not be reached in this instance. When negotiating, be clear with the patient what you can and cannot do for them, and your bottom line. Use your active listening to the maximum – summarise, clarify, reframe, and check. Try to empathise even when this may be difficult. Stay credible, honest, and listen to their perspective. If necessary, ask for time to think. Try not to be punitive, make assumptions, or be intimidated into making unwise or hasty decisions.

There may be occasions when, despite your best efforts, anger cannot be successfully managed. Watch for signs of escalation – a change in the speed or tone of voice, including going quiet or unresponsive, or the use of abusive words, or increasingly intimidating body language. When there seems to be a real threat of physical violence, avoid confrontation at all costs – your physical safety is of paramount importance. If possible, move away and get help. If you have a panic button, press it.

For any incident involving an angry person, make thorough notes afterwards, ensuring you have an accurate record of what was said by you both. As with any difficult consultation, ensure you "housekeep" – don't try to carry on with the day without giving yourself time to decompress and regroup. Debriefing with colleagues in the immediate aftermath can be very beneficial. You should also consider raising a learning event to be discussed at a team meeting later. (If you have a management role yourself, always support any colleagues who might have encountered aggression. This is both a moral suggestion and a practical one. If you do not provide such support, soon there will not be many colleagues left.)

Somatisation/Medically Unexplained Symptoms

A commonly encountered difficulty is the patient who attends repeatedly with physical symptoms that are unclassifiable by an increasingly investigative clinician. We consider these scenarios in two broad groups. One is somatisation, the experience of physical symptoms that reflect psychological or emotional distress. René Descartes, the 17th-century French philosopher, has had an enduring but unhelpful influence on (particularly) Western culture, bequeathing us a dualistic view of human beings as having two separate, unrelated aspects: a mind and a body. In fact, we are single biological organisms and the physical, cognitive, psychological, social, and emotional aspects of our lives are indivisibly entwined, affecting and being affected by each other in myriad ways.

People vary in the way they experience stress, anxiety, depression, or adversity. Some locate these firmly as mental states, others experience them as purely physical symptoms, and many are a mixture. If somatisation is the tendency to experience physical symptoms as part of psychological and emotional responses, then the process by which these are turned into disease by biologically trained clinicians might be termed medicalisation. A medicalising clinician and a somatising patient are a bad combination.

Most people have episodes involving physical complaints that are not explained by organic disease. Low-grade somatisation is common, especially in primary care. Somatisation is also quite commonly seen in children. People with learning disabilities or personality disorders may be especially prone.

The somatisation process can be aided and abetted by clinicians strenuously trying to make sense of physical complaints, and then creating a label which imprints into the patient's mind and is very difficult to dispel. The problem for clinicians in this context is that if patients keep presenting, we will eventually do something. This could be a test, which will lead to a procedure, which can lead to an operation, which can lead to a complication, which in turn will reinforce the patient's health-seeking behaviour.

So, what can we do about this? Quite frequently we will need to conduct some form of physical evaluation – the patient with the racing heart, sweating, and insomnia, for example, will need their blood pressure taken, their chest auscultated, some basic bloods taken and quite possibly an ECG (as well as a review of their medication). A helpful strategy at the outset is to enquire about life circumstances in tandem, emphasising that you are keeping an open mind but that you are undertaking the tests to rule out certain medical conditions. If they come back normal, as you expect, it will be important to consider further whether what they're experiencing is their body's response to stress or strain. Always ensure you acknowledge that the symptoms they're experiencing are real – they are not "imagining" them, nor are they "all in their head". Make links to everyday experiences – the diarrhoea or nausea, dry mouth or racing heart that most people remember prior to taking an important exam, or when going on a first date, or before the bungee-jumping they did on holiday. By taking an explicitly biopsychosocial approach from the get-go, we can start to introduce patients to the concept of somatisation.

This may prove successful when encountering low-grade somatisation, but at the most extreme end of the spectrum – where labels such as "somatic symptom disorder" or "health anxiety" might apply – patients may prove fixated on a biomedical diagnosis. In less enlightened times, they were referred to as "heartsink" or "fat folder" patients, indicating their effect on the clinicians caring for them, and the volume of notes accumulated during exhaustive attempts at trying to do so.

Strategies for Managing Somatically Fixated Patients

Remember conflicting agendas. A somatically fixated patient's agenda will be to find a biomedical diagnosis to explain their symptoms. Yours most broadly should be to help them. Take care that your agenda doesn't get narrowed purely into pursuing a diagnosis, or simply to "proving" there isn't one – neither of these is likely to be that helpful.

Getting ICE out in the open is vital, so that if a specific diagnosis is feared – bowel cancer, for example – a shared plan to address this with minimally invasive investigation might be agreed. A study reported in the *British Journal of General Practice* (Nijrolder et al., 2009) showed that the strongest predictor of poor outcome in patients presenting with "tired all the time" was their expectation of chronicity. Provisional reassurance that much medically unexplained fatigue spontaneously remits over time, coupled with an undertaking to follow up at intervals to keep them under review, can be therapeutically valuable.

Diaries and other methods of self-recording may produce insight and linkage between events and symptoms. Psychologists call this the *de-fusion of the organic versus the functional*, and they use strategies to help patients "reattribute" their explanations for ill health. These strategies include emphasising the role of anxiety in muscular tension, pain, and hyperventilation, the effect of depression on pain thresholds, and the vicious circle of chronic pain and psychological distress. Use reflection to try to aid de-fusion. "I know you've not been feeling well this past year. There have been the tummy pains, the headaches, the fatigue. Do you think there could be something worrying you underneath all this? It's something we commonly see".

Use the disease-based biomedical model with care. Although we all need to be good diagnosticians, good efficient clinical practice demands balances – most headaches do not warrant brain imaging. And while we have an extensive pharmacopoeia, chronic pain rarely responds well to analgesic drugs and may be compounded by them. We must be aware of the danger of medicalisation and the very real iatrogenic harm that can result.

Be on your guard against behaviour that can come across as manipulative. Often individuals are labelled as "manipulative" unfairly when they are simply acting in a way consistent with their own concerns and expectations in the face of resistance and lack of empathy from health professionals. It is essential to spot this process and attempt to address it directly rather than simply say it is the patient's problem.

GPs and other clinicians in primary care must think hard about referral. We still believe that one of the GP's primary duties is to protect his or her patients from unnecessary hospital medicine. Hospital medicine is almost exclusively biomedical; patients must be diagnosed thoroughly, and possible causes ruled out. Once a somatising patient gets to outpatients the die is cast – investigation is coming with all that might entail. The fixation with the symptoms will be intensified and the self-reinforcing loop encouraged. The modern hospital's ability to dig up some minor disorder which is essentially irrelevant, and to overtreat it, is formidable. There is also the danger that, not unreasonably, the patient may be asked to return repeatedly on the grounds that something may have been overlooked (or harried clinicians might use this as a strategy to end consultations). Both of these situations will probably lead the patient to conclude that they were right, and that there is something wrong with their health. If referral is made, the reasons should be set out explicitly, and the clinician who accepts the referral should, whenever possible, keep within the mandate of the referral letter.

Try to limit the number of clinicians involved with a particular patient as much as possible. The more there are, the greater the chance of medicalisation. Regular – for example, monthly – appointments with a specified clinician can be an effective strategy for reducing medicalisation by ensuring the patient feels they are being "held" by the practice. Continuity of care is especially powerful in developing a safe and ideally increasingly biopsychosocial understanding of the problems. Keep good records. Other clinicians who might be involved need to know what your plans are, whether you fear a somatising/medicalising process is happening to the patient, and your strategies for preventing harm. This can be challenging in this age of patient access to records. Already this is changing the way that we document our notes and impressions. Always write your notes as if your patient will be reading them and ensure they are accurate and reflect the conversations you have had. Care is needed when recording information you feel may be counterproductive or harmful for your patient to read, especially if from a third party or regarding a safeguarding concern – in these circumstances it can be appropriate to mark this information so that it cannot be viewed by the patient, but this should always be justifiable.

Remember that somatisation is frequently associated with anxiety and/or depression (whether that be cause, effect, or both). A carefully negotiated trial of treatment may be achievable with even the most somatically focused patient – or it may be possible to broker an agreement to consult with a psychologist, if the patient is able to entertain the possibility of somatisation as an explanation for their experiences.

Try to avoid giving too much advice. Any advice should be specific (i.e. to give a new approach to the problem), and it should be realistically tailored to the individual patient. Be alert to "duck shooting" – if every suggestion you make is "shot down" with reasons why it won't work/can't be done, you have not got a shared understanding. Reflect that back to the patient, go back to the drawing board, and try again. Encourage the patient's internal search and encourage them to find their own solutions and alternative strategies.

While somatisation is to a certain extent "medically explained" (at least in the clinician's mind), a second group of patients might better be thought of as having "medically unexplained physical symptoms" (MUPS). There are a number of syndromes which are well described but currently have no recognised biomedical pathophysiology – conditions like ME/CFS, fibromyalgia, POTS, Long Covid, as well as patients with less succinctly classified clusters of symptoms.

Many of the same pitfalls that can arise in trying to manage somatisation can also apply to these patients – medicalisation, dismissal as "manipulative", "doctor shopping". We don't propose a detailed discussion in this book about these syndromes, other than to make a plea for medical humility. Remember that at any point in medical history, knowledge is only ever provisional and quite often proves to be wrong – peptic ulcer disease used to be managed surgically, for example. Patients with symptoms and disabilities that we cannot account for within our current paradigm are nevertheless fellow human beings suffering ill-health, and we can offer support and care even if we don't currently understand the underlying processes. Many of the approaches to somatising patients can be of value when trying to help someone with MUPS, including trying to minimise medicalisation and iatrogenic harm. In addition, techniques such as motivational interviewing may help facilitate a change in the patient's experience.

Useful questions here are as follows:

- What would you most like to talk about?
- How important is it to change …?
- How might things be different if …?
- How confident do you feel about changing …?

Helping people quantify and rate things can help them seem more manageable for you both. Someone who experiences chronic pain described as "terrible", which dominates their life, may, on further exploration, actually have times in the day where the pain is only 5/10 and they can get out to walk the dog. Perhaps the worst time is the evening when they are tired, and the pain goes up to 9/10, and this could be the area for your initial focus. Pain teams often have no better treatments than anyone else but are experts in this approach and see results. In the face of seemingly insurmountable problems, helping the patient to set more manageable goals can be useful.

Working in MDTs

Teamworking is a key part of functioning within a cohesive health service (or the aspiration of one anyway) and has long been part of the role of all clinicians in both primary and secondary care. However, this is now going further than ever before, and in primary care the development of larger, at-scale organisations has produced a diversification of the traditional patient-facing workforce to match that in hospitals, or even exceed it.

Secondary care specialist nurses and primary care advanced nurse practitioners have been working independently alongside doctors for years. A change more recently in some clinical scenarios has led to the traditional history taking being performed not by a doctor, but by another healthcare professional such as a junior nurse, a physician assistant, or healthcare assistant. The doctor is only called in for the examination and management stage of the consultation, and sometimes not at all. This is in some ways analogous to the long-standing hospital model of clerking, where the resident doctor takes the history and performs the examination, and presents to the senior colleague who fills in any gaps and then comes up with the management plan, but the difference here is that the doctor is working with non-doctor colleagues.

If you are the doctor working in these models, you need to recognise the impact on your ability to manage your patient that having the history told to you by someone else has. You are relying on someone else's ability to elicit the patient's ideas, concerns, and expectations appropriately, and ensuring that a shared understanding has been reached.

This model's obvious benefits are the reduced time that a doctor needs to spend with a patient, and therefore the greater number of patients that can be seen and managed. There are not enough doctors in the system, and allied health professionals are a way of increasing much-needed capacity for managing demand within the NHS. We are having to evolve to survive, and as has been seen many times in history, it is the rush of innovation under pressure that leads to systemic advances and progress.

The concern is that this model leads to a fragmentation of the consultation, with all the inherent risks involved. It is less likely that a patient will feel able to open up about difficult subjects or build a rapport with their health professional that enables true sharing of understanding and decision-making. Continuity reduces, and with it the knowledge of a particular patient and the ability to place them in their own context. We feel it is vitally important to not lose sight of the individual patient in the packed surgery or outpatient clinic. We must be wary of focusing solely on the short-term gains of increasing capacity and forgetting the long-term goal: *that to properly share understanding and decision-making with a patient is more likely to lead them to engage, follow medical advice and treatment, and take responsibility for their own health.*

When working as part of a team, it is not just communication with the patient that is important, but communication within the team as well. Many of the principles of effective listening and communication are just as important when dealing with our colleagues as with our patients. Teams that communicate well are inevitably more effective.

A Final Thought

The health system is changing, and more quickly over the last decade than in the several that came before. The structure of the system in which care is provided is altering, and the routes that patients take through the system are varied. New pathways abound, often accessed by a mountainous catalogue of proformas and referral criteria, with varying levels of service and resource across the country. Is it any wonder our patients often arrive at our doors confused and a little lost?

General practice in particular is currently undergoing something of a seismic shift as many of us change from traditional small and independent practices to larger at-scale organisations, either through choice or necessity. Whether this is a good thing or not is not for us to say, but it will inevitably impact on the environment in which we see our patients, and we must be aware of that. Continuity of care is at threat, although we hope that if GPs are aware enough of the risks, these can be mitigated by good consulting and by influencing system design. We all have various opinions on the direction of travel in the current NHS system. The inevitable fallout of a collapsing social care system is wreaking havoc with community services and hospital capacity alike. Resources are scarce and often misdirected, and policy changes on political whim and agenda. Politics is far outside our remit here, but to ignore the impact of major large-scale and system-wide change on the dynamics of the clinician–patient consultation would be both wishful thinking and naïve.

References

Gross J et al. Intensive care: Balancing risk and benefit to guide informed decisions. *BMJ*. 2018;363:k4135.

Nijrolder I, van der Windt D, van der Horst H. Prediction of outcome in patients presenting with fatigue in primary care. *Br J Gen Pract*. 2009;59(561):e101–e109.

Pitkethly M et al. Recordings or summaries of consultations for people with cancer. *Cochrane Database Syst Rev*. 2008 Jul 16:(3):CD001539. doi: 10.1002/14651858.CD001539.pub2

CHAPTER

8

Wider Communication and Ethical Issues

Our most cruel failure in how we treat the sick and the aged is the failure to recognise that they have priorities beyond merely being safe and living longer.

Atul Gawande

- Try and see the patient in front of you as an individual.
- True, informed consent requires effort.
- Information will mean different things to different patients.

"Whole Patient Medicine"

What is going on when a patient consults a clinician?

On the face of it, the answer appears straightforward. The patient has an illness, and they hope or expect that the clinician will be able to help. Intrinsic to that are faith in the clinician's expertise, and trust that the clinician will do their best for them. The clinician's responsibilities are clear. They have a duty to make the care of that individual patient their first concern. That duty has many facets, including ensuring that any advice and treatment they offer

DOI: 10.1201/9781003652137-8

is appropriate and up to date, and that they work within the limits of their competence.

So far so good, but let's dive a little deeper. Only then will we appreciate how fundamental skilled communication is to proper ethical practice.

First, how does the clinician decide what advice and treatment to offer? That flows from making a diagnosis – in short, how to understand the patient's illness (the symptoms they're experiencing, the effects they are having on them). Within Western medicine, there are two principal diagnostic approaches, the "medical model" and the "biopsychosocial" one. It's important to understand the difference. The medical model essentially views the human being as a machine – admittedly a fiendishly complex one – that can go wrong in a finite number of comprehensible ways, which we call diseases. So, a painful knee might be due to a wide range of pathologies. The history of onset, the pattern of symptoms, the examination findings and investigations are all clues in deciding which one – and therefore what advice and treatment to offer.

Let's say the medical model leads to a diagnosis of osteoarthritis. The clinician might prescribe painkillers, offer a steroid injection, refer for physiotherapy, or even for surgery. But what if the patient is able to manage the symptoms but is fearful they might mean an end to their lifelong passion for running and the social life that revolves around their running club? If the clinician elicited those psychosocial ideas and concerns, they could explain that, although OA is commonly referred to as "wear and tear", that is a misnomer. The best thing the patient can do would be to continue exercising, maintaining their fitness, and keeping their musculature strong.

It's easy to see how that kind of good communication improves outcomes, but surely it wouldn't be *unethical* to have failed to establish that? Well, it very easily could. If the patient is worried about the future and the clinician instead assumes they simply want something to relieve pain, the patient may embark on an unwarranted treatment for the wrong reasons – assuming that, if the clinician recommended it, it must be going to improve their prognosis. At the very least, that would be poor practice, and in the worst case – where a patient suffered a side effect, for instance – there could be avoidable harm. Then there is the impact on other patients. Resources consumed by treating one person are not available for others.

Excellent communication is foundational to ethical practice, and unaddressed assumptions are its antithesis.

What about a situation where the medical model – the "bio" in biopsychosocial – is wholly inadequate? There are myriad conditions as we discussed in the last chapter – IBS, non-epileptic attack disorder (NEAD), ME/CFS, fibromyalgia, Long Covid, to name but a few – where we currently have a very incomplete understanding of the disease mechanisms, and few if any effective treatments. Clinicians bound in the medical model will soon discover the limits of their ability to understand and help these patients. They will often load them with drugs that have little or no chance of benefit and substantial risk of harm, again leading to unethical practice. And the clinician may become averse to seeing the patient's name on the appointment screen, feeling uncomfortable that they have nothing further to offer. This can result in consultations that leave a patient feeling dismissed, unsupported, or not cared for. But these are people experiencing troubling symptoms just like someone with an osteoarthritic knee. Approaching them as unique individuals and eliciting the psychosocial dimensions of their illness enables clinicians to try to improve their suffering even though our biological understanding is incomplete (explaining our limitations can be an important first step).

There is an inherent conflict between the reductionist, disease-based medical model and the genuinely biopsychosocial model that emphasises unwellness or maladaptation of a person in the context of their family, relationships, and society. Avoiding the worst excesses of this conflict requires clinicians to see their patients as individuals and to consider the whole person and their medical problems in an embracing rather than exclusive style. This is more natural for GPs and more difficult for the hospital specialist. For any clinician, it becomes more possible with continuity of care. With the rise of subspecialisation, hospital clinics overall take a narrower and narrower view. Multi-morbid patients end up under the care of many different teams, each working within their silo. Quite aside from the numbers of hospital trips, investigations, procedures, and medications that this entails, patients become increasingly confused as to how to live with and manage their multiple medical problems. This is an ethical reason for regretting the demise of the generalist in hospitals. The medical generalist in the community – the GP – will often be the one professional able to help these patients achieve holistic outcomes amid the confusion – an ethical reason to regret the currently dwindling numbers of doctors in primary care.

Informed Consent

We've seen how good communication skills are central to a clinician developing the fullest possible understanding of their patient's illness – a holistic or biopsychosocial diagnosis. This diagnosis will usually lead to advice and treatment (which should always include the option of doing nothing). Here, too, there are important ethical dimensions.

Most people will be aware of the concept of consent. For much of medical history, this consisted in a doctor saying, "In my opinion, this is what should be done" and the patient going along with it. The content of any explanation was entirely at the doctor's discretion. Hippocrates' famous but rather weird oath makes no reference at all to a doctor's duty to converse with patients. Plato, in several of his writings, stated quite categorically that doctors had a right to employ lies for good and noble purposes. In the eighteenth and nineteenth centuries, a few isolated luminaries suggested educating and involving patients. John Gregory, Professor of Medicine at Edinburgh, was a notable example, and Benjamin Rush, a famous American contemporary of Gregory, held similar views but, like Gregory, favoured deception whenever enlightenment was not equal to the task.

In the latter half of the twentieth century, this approach began to be supplanted by a transatlantic concept, that of *informed* consent, first mentioned in a California Supreme Court judgment in 1957. For truly ethical practice, a patient should be aware of all options open to them for treating their illness (including doing nothing), the likely outcomes of each, the chances of harm with each scenario, and what that harm might mean.

The first challenge is how much information is it reasonable and useful for a clinician to impart. Surgeons have generally become very comprehensive: it is usual for letters to patients to detail long lists of every complication recognised to arise from any proposed operation, including vanishingly rare ones. Quite what patients make of these litanies of offputtingly scary scenarios is debatable, and this mode of informed consent may be more to do with professional protection than true patient engagement. Physicians are typically at the opposite end of the spectrum. Most prescriptions for new pharmaceuticals will come with scant discussion of potential side effects, and certainly of few very rare serious ones. (There are exceptions, which are often bizarre and idiosyncratic, such as the warnings routinely dispensed about Fournier's gangrene to anyone embarking on SGLT-2 treatment.)

Given that failed communication about risks of treatment may very well become legal matters, one might expect the law to give some guidance on what truly informed consent looks like. When Peter wrote the first edition of this book, English case law governing informed consent was based on what was known as the Bolam test. In essence, this held that it was up to the doctor to determine what constituted reasonable information to impart when obtaining consent, and provided a good number of peers would agree with what the doctor had done, consent would be deemed to have been properly informed.

However, between the seventh and eighth editions of this book appearing, UK law was updated. *Montgomery v. Lanarkshire Health Board* [2015] UKSC 11 came before the Supreme Court in 2015 and has had a highly significant impact. A woman gave birth to a baby boy, sadly born with severe disabilities due to complications in labour. The mother was of small stature and suffered from insulin-dependent diabetes mellitus, and the delivery of her baby was complicated by large foetal size and shoulder dystocia. The mother had raised concerns antenatally and during labour about the safety of delivering her baby vaginally but had not asked about exact risks. The mother was not informed of the risk of shoulder dystocia prior to or during her labour because her consultant felt that to do so would lead her to opt for a caesarean section, which the consultant felt was not in her best interests. The mother brought the case to court claiming negligence on the grounds that, had she been aware of the risk, she would have asked for an elective caesarean section delivery, and her son would have been born unharmed. The Montgomery case concluded with the following (paragraphs 87 and 88):

> *An adult person of sound mind is entitled to decide which, if any, of the available forms of treatment to undergo .... The doctor is therefore under a duty to take reasonable care to ensure that the patient is aware of any material risks involved in any recommended treatment, and of any reasonable alternative or variant treatments. The test of materiality is whether, in the circumstances of the particular case, a reasonable person in the patient's position would be likely to attach significance to the risk, or the doctor is or should reasonably be aware that the particular patient would be likely to attach significance to it.*
>
> *The doctor is however entitled to withhold from the patient information as to a risk if he reasonably considers that its disclosure would be seriously detrimental to the patient's health. The doctor is also excused from conferring with the patient in circumstances of necessity, as for example where the patient requires treatment urgently but is unconscious or otherwise unable to make a decision.*

The Montgomery judgment has replaced the Bolam test as the legal basis of the duties of gaining informed consent. It puts emphasis on what significance patients would attach to a given risk and places a duty on a clinician to ensure they are aware of factors particular to them as an individual that might affect what information should be given.

Even these updated legal frameworks leave considerable room for doubt over how much clinicians should be expected to tell patients when seeking informed consent. The American researchers, Greenfield et al. (1985), turned this conundrum on its head. They asked themselves the question: if doctors do not inform patients well enough, what will happen if we teach patients to ask searching questions of their doctors and to negotiate decisions relating to their own care? They took three groups of patients from a California hospital – people with peptic ulcers, people with high blood pressure, and people with diabetes. Using a randomised technique, they split each group into two and trained one half to ask appropriate questions and negotiate decisions. They then measured outcomes. So, what happened? Lo and behold, in the intervention groups the blood sugar level improved significantly, the blood pressure dropped significantly, ulcers improved more quickly, and the patients were happier and liked the involvement. If these results had been achieved with a new medication then the pharmaceutical companies would have been ecstatic, but all that was in fact needed was some additional two-way communication. There is now a substantial body of evidence that such approaches to "patient activation" are associated with improved health outcomes and patient experience, and probably reduced costs across a wide range of health conditions (Greene et al., 2015), with no adverse impact on consultation time (Bruch, 2024).

The fact that informed consent is now such a major issue is good for patients, as they are offered more information than ever before. Surgeries overflow with leaflets on every conceivable subject, hospital outpatient departments have printed sheets on most known diseases and procedures, but the main driver of this change has been the internet. There is more medical information readily available online than we could ever know, and patients are increasingly more curious and more inclined to do their own research before presenting to a professional. This means that patients can enter the consultation with specific ideas, concerns, and expectations. GPs are now often seen as the enabler, or conduit, to the investigations or treatments that the patient already knows (or thinks they know) that they need. Equally, the internet is also very good at generating worst-case scenarios (any symptom you can think of could be attributable to cancer) but hopeless at context. Clinicians need to be prepared for how different the consultation can be with a very informed patient, who will sometimes know an awful lot more about a specific condition than the clinician does, yet who may also be highly anxious because they lack the experience to put their symptoms into context. These are challenges that can make it easier to lose track of the patient behind the opinions. As ever, good communication skills are the antidote.

Shared Decision-Making

The real crux of the whole informed consent debate is that to obtain true informed consent requires the achievement of a *shared understanding and a shared management plan* – usually shorthanded as *shared decision-making*. This further implies that the patient's beliefs should be known, and their understanding checked effectively. The ethical imperative behind achieving a shared understanding is respect for the individual. There has long been a tacit assumption that consent can never be truly informed, so that it is for clinicians to determine what is in the patient's best interest. However, health is mainly the subjective experience of an individual and is made up of highly personal beliefs, feelings, and experiences. It follows that, when helped by clinicians to achieve a comprehension of the risks and benefits of various treatments, it is patients and only patients who can really determine which therapy will help them to achieve their most important health goals.

Most consent is still a long way from being informed. The internet contains information ranging from medical fact and accepted practice to myth, supposition, and downright falsehood. Most leaflets, while factual, are not very good; some are very poor, and some make no sense at all. The moral here is that useful information presented in an inaccessible way is useless information. Information will mean different things to different patients depending on their health understanding, and what is readily understandable to one will be incomprehensible to another. A signature of consent may just mean that the patient trusts the clinician, not that they genuinely understand what is to be done to them and what risks there may be. Clinicians are still very influential people, and we must use this influence with care.

True consent is increasingly regarded as a right, and if this right is seen to be denied or infringed, litigation ensues more and more frequently. Until very recently, there was a prevailing attitude that people in hospital would be unable and unwilling to engage in any discussion about their treatment or future pathway. Of course, it now seems obvious to most that this is nonsense. In fact, patients become less anxious if they are adequately informed about major surgical procedures, nasty invasive tests, unpleasant treatments, and dangerous drugs. Many will have a clear wish to participate in shared decision-making and, in many instances, this will lead to a better therapeutic partnership and outcome. Clinicians need to do all they can to ensure patients can meaningfully participate in their care, including, where appropriate, directing changes to their treatment or declining it altogether.

The issue of capacity is obviously key here. Where people lack capacity to consent for any reason, the Mental Capacity Act (MCA) 2005 applies, and treatment of any condition may be given in their best interests. This is always a tricky area. The MCA enshrines the principle of an assumption of capacity. This suggests that we ought not to go looking too deeply for a lack of capacity where it is not obvious. However, many people probably understand considerably less than required to comprehend the treatments we propose. Then there is the issue of making unwise choices: people with capacity are allowed to make eccentric decisions.

Here are a few statements from the NHS Constitution (2023) on this topic:

You have the right to accept or refuse treatment that is offered to you, and not to be given any physical examination or treatment unless you have given valid consent. If you do not have the capacity to do so, consent must be obtained from a person legally able to act on your behalf, or the treatment must be in your best interests.

You have the right to be given information about the test and treatment options available to you, what they involve and their risks and benefits.

It may be that informed consent is already an outmoded concept, and that instead patients should be encouraged to actively request a particular form of treatment after having been adequately informed of the options. This request shifts the onus onto the patient – the consumers of healthcare take responsibility for their choice. This behaviour was unheard of when Peter wrote the first edition of this book in 1994. Our role as clinicians is changing from informer to interpreter, so we need to get used to it. The future is now.

Anticipatory Health Measures

We began this chapter thinking about what goes on when a patient with an illness consults a clinician. We've seen how good communication is fundamental to ethical practice. Now let's consider something very different and increasingly common: situations in which it is the *clinician* (or the health service, or even the government) encouraging someone in good health to become a patient.

The broad term to describe these scenarios is "anticipatory health measures" – there isn't a problem now but there might be in the future, and doing something at this stage might lead to better outcomes than would otherwise occur. Anticipatory health measures in the United Kingdom include the established national screening programmes for certain cancers (cervical, breast, bowel), the efforts through NHS Health Checks to assess people for cardiovascular risk factors, as well as initiatives by both the NHS and health charities to heighten people's awareness and anxiety about specific diseases and promote contact with health services that would not otherwise occur.

Amid this cacophony of anticipatory health measures, the same principles of shared decision-making and informed consent apply. So, what is different about these scenarios, and what role do communication skills play in ensuring ethical practice is maintained?

The fundamental question is: Whose agenda is it? A patient deciding to consult a clinician is very obviously addressing their own concerns, but anticipatory health measures are far murkier. Ostensibly about improving individual health, they are tightly bound up in population-level considerations. Preventing disease should, in theory at least, reduce health service costs, as should detecting it at an earlier stage when treatment may be cheaper and more effective. Both these aims should keep people fit and economically active for longer, increasing tax revenues and GDP while minimising spending on benefits. All these things are in a government's (and arguably a society's) interest, so considerable effort is invested to ensure cooperation. But populations are comprised of numerous individuals, all of whom have a rightful expectation of genuine involvement in decisions about their health.

So how does a person decide whether to undertake a particular anticipatory health measure? At its most basic, they might do so on trust. If their clinician or the health service is offering it, it must be a good thing, so best to go ahead. A significant problem is that people generally overestimate the likelihood of benefit from a medical intervention, and similarly underestimate the chances of suffering harm (Hoffman, 2015). To give properly informed consent to an anticipatory health measure, they would need accurate information about a host of factors:

- What level of risk applies to me?
- What level of benefit could I expect from taking up this anticipatory measure?
- What are the limitations or disadvantages of the proposed assessments or tests?
- What harms could arise and how likely are they?
- What else might I do and how does that compare?
- What would happen if I did nothing?
- Are there conflicts of interest underpinning this proposed intervention?

We'll come to the question of risk shortly, but first let's look at the balance between benefit and harm. Anticipatory health measures aim to do good by preventing or mitigating a future illness. Broadly speaking, harms arise from overdiagnosis and overtreatment. Considering cancer screening, medicine's ability to detect abnormalities has far outstripped our prognostic capabilities. Many screen-detected tumours will never cause clinical disease, but because in most cases we can't distinguish which could be safely left alone, all get treated – with the attendant potential to cause often substantial harm.

It has been a long and uphill battle to ensure this information is made available to prospective screening participants, in large part because of the conflict between the population and the personal. An Australian study looking into screening for bowel cancer using faecal occult blood (Smith et al., 2010) randomised those with lower educational attainment to receive different levels of additional information about the procedure. The study revealed that those with more information reported that they knew more, made more informed choices, and found the decision easier to make than those who did not receive further information. The surprising finding was that fewer of the educated group decided to take the test. The deeply depressing editorial accompanying this paper suggested that "adherence" might be better achieved by "a policy of informed uptake rather than informed decision making".

This instinct to emphasise the positives and downplay the negatives to promote uptake over informed consent was evident in the literature originally accompanying the breast screening programme in the United Kingdom. Only after a prolonged campaign was the leaflet rewritten in 2013 to better balance benefits with harms (though criticisms remain). Of 200 women going through the 20-year screening programme, only one can expect her life to be "saved", i.e. she will avoid death from breast cancer. One hundred and ninety-six women will derive no benefit and a few of them will experience harm from earlier diagnosis without prognostic advantage. And a further three women will be diagnosed and go through aggressive treatment

– potentially including radiotherapy, chemotherapy, and hormonal blockade, as well as running a higher risk of undergoing mastectomy – entirely unnecessarily.

In another context, this might give rise to searching questions, but as an editorial in the *BMJ* of September 2018 explains,

> *Ironically, even though it causes harm, the effects of overdiagnosis look like benefits. People with disease that is overdiagnosed do well because, by definition, their disease was non-progressive. They are 'cured' when the cure was not necessary in the first place. This creates a cycle that reinforces efforts leading to more overdiagnosis.*
>
> *A screening test that results in substantial overdiagnosis improves survival statistics by diluting the diagnosed pool with many non-progressive cases, which makes screening seem more effective than it is. The spurious rise in incidence makes the case for screening more compelling, thus heightening people's sense of risk – a phenomenon known as the popularity paradox.*
>
> **(Brodersen et al., 2018, k3494)**

A related conundrum to the question of benefit versus harm is that of risk. Most anticipatory health measures are focused on those with a higher risk of the target disease (which improves the cost-benefit calculation) but that's only one side of the coin. To encourage uptake among the healthy population, they must perceive themselves to *be* at risk (why else would you get screened, particularly if in doing so you will suffer embarrassment or discomfort?).

Our perception of risk is highly malleable. Personal experiences, things that have happened to family or friends, articles in magazines or online, awareness-raising campaigns on the part of health charities or the NHS – all affect how vulnerable we feel at any given time. The ways clinicians communicate risk will also influence their patients' decisions about anticipatory health measures, so there is an ethical dimension to this aspect of clinical practice.

This might be subtle and deceptively passive: merely sending a screening invitation under a practice's letterhead implies endorsement. Or we may play a more active part. When it comes to the primary prevention of cardiovascular disease, we routinely deploy risk "calculators" to stratify patients. These churn out numerical answers expressed to two decimal places, endowing what is a crude rule of thumb with an aura of unerring accuracy. And if the risk is above an arbitrary threshold the number is displayed on screen in alarming red, creating the impression of seriousness and urgency. Yet most people deemed "high risk" will never develop cardiovascular disease. And most cases of heart attacks and stroke will arise in people classified as "lower risk".

This becomes evident when one looks at the numbers needed to treat (NNT) or absolute risk reductions (ARR). Drug treatment for stage 1 hypertension, for example, is largely ineffective. Depending on the baseline risk there can be a less than 0.02% chance that medication will benefit an individual in any one year, and treatment fails to prevent most cardiovascular events. Yet how often is a patient with, say, a BP of 155/95 told "Your blood pressure is too high, you'd better take something to control it". If detail is given, it might be in the form of relative risk reduction (RRR), which invariably makes interventions sound much more useful. For the same 0.02% ARR scenario in stage 1 hypertension, how does, "This pill reduces your chance of a heart attack or stroke by up to 12%" sound?

The other side of the ethical imperative to do good is to do no harm. The very marginal benefits of medicating for much raised blood pressure need to be set against the anxiety, medicalisation, side effects, and expense of treatment. Hypertension has reached plague proportions and irrespective of treatment, the diagnosis is associated with an increase in absenteeism, sport is avoided, impotence rates quadruple, and the "hypertensive" person now sees himself or herself differently. This is a label that makes people sick, so clinicians have to do an awful lot of good to make up for it. David Misselbrook, in his excellent book *Thinking about Patients* (2001), suggests that you ask your hypertensive patients three questions:

1 Do you ever wonder if you might be experiencing side effects from your medication?
2 Do you often think about your blood pressure?
3 Does your blood pressure cause you any problems in your day-to-day life?

He found very high levels of anxiety and a feeling of being stigmatised by the label. Try it yourself.

Patients who are well informed will frequently make choices that go against purely population-level thinking. The benefits of stroke prevention by anticoagulation in atrial fibrillation seem clear-cut to most clinicians, but in an American study of a group of patients who were well informed of the pros and cons, a significant proportion decided not to choose the intervention (Yao et al., 2022). Tellingly, rather than celebrating this diversity of shared decision-making outcomes, the authors interpreted their results as demonstrating a need to do more to increase anticoagulant use.

A major problem with communication about risk is the differing frames of reference used by patients and clinicians. Professionals use mathematical concepts such as AAR, RRR, NNT, and NNH (number needed to harm). Patients with varying loci of control see themselves, for very unmathematical reasons, as being high, medium, or low risk, and then use the lottery logic of luck, fate, and destiny to make an individual and unique assessment. If we allow them, our patients will tell us compelling stories to communicate their perspectives. Clinicians, on the other hand, relate statistics but without the persuasive reality and impact of the stories that our patients tell. The burning question that our patient wants to ask is, "Do you really think that taking this tablet for the next 30 years is definitely going to do me more good than harm?" In formulating our answer, it behoves us to reflect on the place we as clinicians are coming from.

The Ethics of the Medical Agenda

This is a complex area that has received too little attention in the past. It is a *sine qua non* of modern medicine that our practice is based on "evidence". The evidence-based medicine movement has grown from small beginnings in the 1990s to dominate every aspect of what clinicians do today. It seems to provide seductive certainties. Guidelines exist for virtually every medical model diagnosis, as well as the assessment and management of the risk factors for major diseases, describing in detail what advice and treatment should be offered. But we should remain humble and alert to the assumptions and biases within this apparently objective frame of reference.

Most medical evidence is derived from reductive science (the gold standard of which is the randomised controlled trial or RCT) which seeks to limit the number of variables in order to address very specific questions. This produces clear answers, certainly, but their applicability to real life, where things are complex and strewn with messy variables, is far from a given.

A related issue concerns multimorbidity and frailty. Most evidence is generated in the context of single diseases, but most real-world patients have several. The patients selected for trials are also typically younger and fitter than the counterparts that clinicians deal with in everyday life. The uncritical application of the evidence generated by these rarefied trials, embodied in the ubiquitous single-disease guidelines that surround us, greatly increases the chances of iatrogenic harm from the polypharmacy that so frequently results.

The production of evidence also costs money – lots of it. Most is paid for by the pharmaceutical and technological industries. Most medical evidence therefore focuses on drugs and the application of technologies, through which corporate profits are to be made. So, when clinicians reach for the "evidence", this is what they find. And there is a profound influence on the prevailing culture. We become unconsciously biased towards technological and pharmaceutical approaches to healthcare – biases many of our patients simply do not share.

There are also the goals that the producers of evidence are most concerned about. All too frequently these are longevity (easy to measure) rather than quality of life (hard). To quote Iona Heath (1999), an eminent GP who worked in Kentish Town, London, and one-time president of the Royal College of General Practitioners:

> *Medical science has valued the simple statistics of longevity above any measures of the quality of life .... Much more work needs to be done to analyse and describe the limitations of biomedical science, the importance of death, and the overwhelming need to incorporate the patients' own values and aspirations into a system of care which is increasingly driven by standardised protocols. We must recognise the tendency for medical science to become totalitarian.*
>
> **(Heath, 1999)**

This totalitarian tendency is, of course, a continuation of the old beneficent paternalism, given added momentum by some new conflicts of interest. Remember the attraction to governments of population-level health interventions? For many years now, general practitioners have had financial incentives under the Quality and Outcomes Framework (QOF) to ensure patients conform to certain centrally dictated approaches to healthcare. The cholesterol debate illustrates this, specifically when looking at the issue of primary prevention of cardiovascular disease. GPs and their teams have become embroiled in target chasing, prescribing ever more tenuously evidenced pharmaceuticals to ever expanding proportions of the adult population at ever lower estimated risk of heart disease and stroke.

Only a small minority of this activity involves shared decision-making and properly informed consent from the patients involved. One of the challenges in trying to practise ethically in these scenarios is the lack of information underlying the assertions made in guidelines. Treatments with very different effect sizes and applicability are promoted indistinguishably. On top of that, just as patients overestimate the chance of benefit from medical interventions, so do doctors (Hoffman and Del Mar, 2017; Treadwell et al., 2020).

An important step towards remedying this was launched by academic and GP Dr Julian Treadwell in 2023. His website, GPEvidence.org – the product of a DPhil in the Nuffield Department of Primary Health Care Sciences at Oxford – is a user-friendly repository of all the data required for informed consent for a whole host of medical interventions. The site illustrates most of its information with Cates plots – those grids of 100 smiling or unhappy faces that aid rapid, impactful visual appreciation of otherwise arcane statistical details – making it an ideal tool to deploy in shared decision-making. (It will also surprise and sometimes shock you how little value there is in many of the things our guidelines push us into. Have a nose round the site, you'll be amazed.)

Use of such tools takes time – both for initial awareness and training, and for deploying during patient consultations – a resource that's under continual pressure in the NHS. The launch of GPEvidence.org also coincides with the production of a small but growing number of patient decision aids that can be used at home. And many more websites featuring, for example, information about breast screening, are reflecting high-quality information about both pros and cons. Perhaps medical totalitarianism can be turned back yet.

That said, when trying to achieve shared decision-making, it is permissible – perhaps even morally obligatory – for a clinician to attempt by negotiation to change the mind of a patient who is making an apparently irrational choice. It is through these genuine negotiations that the clinician and patient can come to a truly shared understanding of the issues in a way that is best suited to maximising the values of both parties. Although the decision-making process is shared, the final decision should usually be that of the patient. There are, however, limits. Sometimes shared understandings cannot be reached, and in these circumstances patients cannot demand we prescribe something, or arrange an investigation, where we believe it to be wholly inappropriate. There is usually a much greyer area where we are persuaded to increase a dose or prescribe something which just might help but we do not honestly believe actually will. But ultimately, shared decision-making is a two-way, not a one-way street.

Where Does All This Leave Us?

It has always seemed to us that one of the ethical hallmarks of good medical communication is a requirement for honesty. There is an imperative for the clinician to seek and confirm understanding in four main areas: first, that the patient is aware that they are an active part of the decision-making process; second, that they are aware of the choices; third, that they are aware of the implications of those choices; and, finally, that they have assimilated enough specific information on the risks and benefits to allow them to make an informed choice.

A good model must be one of *mutual persuasion* by two experts, one on medical matters and the other on their own mind and body. This implies that clinicians must be prepared to allow themselves to be persuaded by their patients away from their first or second choices of action if the patient's argument is effective, convincing and, most importantly, informed. Clinicians are not always going to like this.

The GMC, in abridged highlights from its *Good medical practice* (2026), is unequivocal in its position:

- Provide a good standard of practice and care, and work within your competence.
- Keep your knowledge and skills up to date.
- Respect every patient's dignity and treat them as an individual.
- Listen to patients and work in partnership with them, supporting them to make informed decisions about their care.
- Treat people with respect and help to create a working and training environment that is compassionate, supportive, and fair, where everyone feels safe to ask questions, talk about errors, and raise concerns.
- Act promptly if you think that patient safety or dignity may be seriously compromised.
- Act with honesty and integrity, and be open if things go wrong.
- Protect and promote the health of patients and the public.

- Never unfairly discriminate against patients or colleagues.
- Never abuse patients' trust in you or the public's trust in your profession.

You are personally accountable for your professional practice and must always be prepared to justify your decisions and actions …

Any clinician who wants to be effective must be interested in people and not merely diseases. They must be committed to their patients' welfare, willing to search out their patients' beliefs, and it follows that they must also be willing to listen to whatever problems the patients bring to them. This is an intensely personal form of healthcare, under increasing pressure in the resource-squeezed NHS of today. The treatment of a disease can be largely impersonal, but the care of a patient is entirely personal. We have an ethical duty to keep it that way.

References

Brodersen J. et al. Focusing on overdiagnosis as a driver of too much medicine. *BMJ*. 2018;362:k3494.

Bruch, JD et al. The effects of shared decision making on health outcomes, health care quality, cost, and consultation time: an umbrella review. *Patient Educ Couns*. 2024 Dec:129:108408. doi: 10.1016/j.pec.2024.108408.

Department of Health. *NHS constitution*. London: Department of Health; 2023 Aug 17.

General Medical Council (GMC). *Good medical practice*. London: General Medical Council; 2026.

Greene J et al. When patient activation levels change, health outcomes and costs change, too. *Health Aff (Millwood)*. 2015 Mar;34(3):431–437. doi: 10.1377/hlthaff.2014.0452.

Greenfield S et al. Expanding patient involvement in care: Effects on patient outcomes. *Ann Intern Med*. 1985;102(4):520–528.

Heath I. William Pickles lecture 1999: 'Uncertain clarity': Contradiction, meaning, and hope. *Br J Gen Pract*. 1999;49(445):651–657.

Hoffmann TC, Del Mar C. Patients' expectations of the benefits and harms of treatments, screening, and tests: a systematic review. *JAMA Intern Med*. 2015;175(2):274–286.

Hoffmann TC, Del Mar C. Clinicians' expectations of the benefits and harms of treatments, screening, and tests: a systematic review. *JAMA Intern Med*. 2017;177(3):407–419.

Misselbrook D. *Thinking about Patients*. Newbury: Petroc Press; 2001.

Smith SK et al. A decision aid to support informed choices about bowel cancer screening among adults with low education: Randomised controlled trial. *BMJ*. 2010;341:c5370.

Treadwell JS et al. GPs' understanding of the benefits and harms of treatments for long-term conditions: an online survey. *BJGP Open* 2020;4(1):bjgpopen20X101016.
Yao C et al. Exploring clinician perspectives on patients with atrial fibrillation who are not prescribed anticoagulation therapy. https://doi.org/10.1016/j.pecinn.2022.100062.

CHAPTER

9

Final Thoughts on Mattering

We hope that over the course of reading this book, whether you have skimmed the salient points or read all the detail, you will appreciate why writing this updated version of *The Doctor's Communication Handbook* (*DCH*) mattered to us. Between the two of us, we have decades of experience of being doctors, working in hospitals across multiple specialities, followed by the majority of our careers in general practice. As practising GPs, we live every day in the world of consultations, some with new and some with familiar patients, every time looking to establish a shared understanding of why that patient has come to see us and what matters to them, to enable us to work together to achieve a genuinely therapeutic outcome. This stuff matters to us because we have the lived experience of seeing it make a difference time and time again, both to our patients and to us.

Not only are we GPs, but we have also, like everyone, had need to visit a GP surgery or hospital ourselves, either for our own health or that of our loved ones. We have experienced first-hand the genuine difference a clinician can make when they choose to listen and understand, rather than adopt a standardised, formulaic approach to the problem at hand. We perhaps have more insight than the typical patient into how a consultation is conducted, and are therefore able to recognise the skill, empathy, and interest shown by clinicians who care what matters, because we know the attitude it demonstrates in them. They are someone that, no matter how pressured or busy, knows that what matters to the patient in front of them is the key to working out how to understand them, and therefore help them, most efficiently and effectively.

DOI: 10.1201/9781003652137-9

By bringing *DCH* up to date with this edition, we have explored how the landscape of UK medicine has changed in the intervening six years since the last, and the ways clinicians have adapted to a faster-paced period of change than any of us have experienced before. We have looked at the impact of these changes on how we consult, where we consult, and whom we can consult with. We can embrace change, but with eyes open to the consequences on our consultations, we can also mitigate the negative impacts. This allows us to not lose sight of what matters the most to us and our patients, whether for a single consultation or a lifetime of care.

We also hope this book can add to the growing number of voices championing continuity of care as a model which must not be lost from UK general practice. Continuity can exist in many shapes and forms, but we must protect and promote the ability for a patient to have continuity with their clinician. We have seen throughout this book how continuity improves patient outcomes and how it also makes our job more effective. Continuity of care is why many of us move to a career in general practice, drawn by the ability to get to know our patients, to understand what matters to them, and to be able to build a genuinely therapeutic relationship over time. If we lose that continuity, we will lose much more than most people realise. Healthcare that shifts to a transactional, access-first, one-size-fits-all approach will be an infinitely poorer place to be cared for and to work in. We can only hope that those who wield power and control within the NHS recognise this before it is lost.

What mattered to Peter when he first wrote *DCH* matters just as much to us today. While *DCH* has over time shifted from an exam-focused text to more of a guidebook for clinicians of all stages in their careers, we hope that this is still a useful text for those just embarking on the early steps of a clinical career. The appendix contains more technical, practical content for those to whom this is relevant.

Our final thought is the hope that you finish this book agreeing that its message matters to you too.

Francesca Frame
Phil Whitaker
2026

Appendix

As we have mentioned, *The Doctor's Communication Handbook* (*DCH*) began life partly as a guide for GP registrars preparing for the video examination component of the MRCGP in the 1990s. Much has changed over the years since the first edition. The concept of ICE has permeated undergraduate medical education, and all doctors graduating from UK medical schools will now be familiar with the importance of good communication and consultation skills and should have at least a basic level of competence. The curricula for every postgraduate training programme for general practice should build on and refine these skills further.

However, although communication and consultation skills are important to every branch of medicine, their development during postgraduate training for doctors in other specialties – and for clinicians training in professions allied to medicine, who conduct increasing numbers of consultations with patients in today's multidisciplinary NHS – remains distinctly patchy (NHS England, 2021). And, as we described in earlier chapters, even where clinicians have a good grounding in the concept of ICE, it is all too often treated as a "tick box" exercise of peripheral importance.

In this latest edition of *DCH*, we have remained faithful to the trajectory followed by its forebears – evolving as a handbook for the practice of patient-centred medicine, which we have updated to reflect the present day. While we have retained some discussion of techniques in the main body of the text, we have removed a lot of the material left over from *DCH*'s origins as an exam guide. For some of our current readership, a more detailed description of techniques may be of interest and use, so we have compiled this material into an appendix to the main book. This, by nature of our book's history and our own experience, is most suited to medical training, but the techniques contained here would be of use to all clinicians.

History Taking

To consult well, you need to be in the right mood, so the first step is to prepare yourself. You must try to generate some enthusiasm and curiosity for the coming encounter. This might be the umpteenth consultation of the day for you, but always remember: for your patient this is likely to be a unique moment and it may well be freighted with importance.

What follows is not the same as the traditional method of history taking. In some ways it amounts to the same thing, but it is a better method. The concepts are rooted in the discussions in the previous chapters, and the model works for all patient encounters in whatever setting (with the exception of the highest acuity presentations like major trauma or cardiac arrest).

There are four main headings:

1 Discover the reasons for the patient's attendance:
   a. Understand the patient.
   b. Understand the problem.
2 Share understanding.
3 Share decisions and responsibility.
4 Make effective use of the consultation.

To use an American expression, let us "unpack" each task in turn.

1. Discover the Reason for Attendance

a. Understand the Patient

We hope it is apparent to you that patients do not come to see clinicians because they have liver disease. They come because they perceive that their health has changed, and they have a whole set of beliefs and expectations relating to this change in health. So where should we start? The best bet is usually with the patient.

THE BEGINNING

Beginnings are very important and will affect the course of the whole meeting, so start open, not closed. Try to connect with the human being in front of you. Some of us are better at this than others, but we can all improve – a smile, an individual greeting in the waiting room, perhaps some easy social banter based on previous consultations, a little bit of personal warmth, and good eye contact.

Avoid the standard opening of "Hello, what can I do for you?" as this is controlling; it implies an action. You may think that this is nit-picking but do experiment with the effects of various opening gambits – what about a simple, "How can I help?" As with chess, you can win or lose the consultation in the first few exchanges.

LISTEN TO THE PATIENT DESCRIBING THE REASONS FOR ATTENDING

Remember William Osler's dictum to listen to the patient because they are trying to tell you the diagnosis. The simplest way to do this is to let the patient talk, actively encourage their contribution to the consultation, and watch them all the time. Try not to interrupt. Research shows that most patients manage to divulge the reasons for their attendance in under a minute (Danczak, 2015). Use your perceptive faculties to hear what they are saying and try to pick up the message behind the message. Pay particular attention to the very first sentence or two they say: you'll be surprised how often you can look back and see that they contained the essence of what the consultation proved to be about.

Letting the patient have a minute or two of relatively uninterrupted speech at the beginning of a consultation often *saves time*. This may be counterintuitive, but it is true. The reasons why letting the patient talk can save time are related first to the patient's agenda and also to yours. The patient, and only the patient, knows the reasons they have come to see you. If you start on your agenda too soon you may never discover what the patient actually wants to know. You may spend precious minutes testing for and explaining cubital tunnel syndrome, but never assure them that you have considered and discounted their fear that they have multiple sclerosis.

The point about you starting on your agenda too soon is significant. It is well documented that we make hypotheses very early on in a consultation – usually in the first 30 seconds, sometimes even earlier. Once you have made a hypothesis, all your energies are channelled towards proving that hypothesis (that pesky *confirmation bias* again). There follows a rapid-fire series of clinical, closed questions directed towards that end, to the exclusion of a broader picture. Another hypothesis will only arise if your clinical search is sterile, or you actively engage your effortful system 2 thinking to search for alternatives. We can be very bad at falling into this trap; some do not even generate differential diagnoses in their head, but leap to the first diagnosis which suggests itself and ask questions which confirm that. You will gain so much more valuable information by consciously delaying making your first hypothesis for, say, just one minute. Try it. It is hard to do at first but very rewarding.

Establishing your patient's agenda early on also allows you to negotiate the use of time – to agree on what will be dealt with now and what can be left for another day. This is a very important skill to learn early in your career, as it can save so much time and prevent so much unnecessary stress.

KEEPING OPEN

Concentrate on asking *open* questions. They are useful for finding out about patients' beliefs, as such questions cannot be answered with a simple yes or no. For example, "Tell me about …", "What is it like?" and so on. You can try making statements which are also good questions. For example, "I was wondering whether …", "Sometimes I find …", "It occurred to me that …", "I've known cases where …", "I had a patient once …", and so on.

The history taking that you have laboriously learned teaches you to ask closed questions, which are useful for obtaining and classifying facts, and for pattern recognition. They are not helpful for eliciting beliefs and feelings, as they tend to increase doctor control and can only be answered very specifically.

You are now in the swing of things, so give your patient some encouragement, such as "Go on" or "Tell me more", which is the best directive we have ever found – patients always do tell you more. Eye contact and nodding encourage the patient to continue.

PICKING UP ON CUES

Always keep watching your patient, so that you do not miss any cues – signals or unconscious prompts that invite a response. Cues may be simply what is said, or they may be what is *not* said. Picking up on the cues that our patients give us is a skill that we all need to develop. This is the way into the real agenda, and if you miss the opportunity, it may not come again. No clinician can hope to be effective or to derive job satisfaction without developing the ability to use cues.

You do not always have to act on them, but ignoring the patient's cues will mean that you will be less effective. As an example of a verbal cue that is not responded to, the patient may say, "It's my back again", and you only address the present episode, without exploring the previous ones implicit in the cue. A patient with headaches may say, "My husband thought I ought to come and see you about these headaches", inviting a response to discuss her husband's concerns. Or, to go back to your consultation with Mrs Arthur in outpatients, you ask, "Is there anything else worrying you?" to which she replies, "Er ... no, I don't think so", while dropping her gaze and nervously fiddling with her handbag. Do you take this denial at face value? You could pick up on her cues and perhaps say, "You do look worried".

You must practise true seeing and hearing. Watch the patient's facial expressions, where they look, and what gestures they make. Do they make eye contact? Watch their posture, muscle tone, and breathing. Do they look anxious, sad, or angry? Think about their dress and their general appearance. Are they fidgety, relaxed, or distant? What might Sherlock Holmes have deduced?

Really listen to them carefully. What does their speech tell you? How are they saying it? Is their speech too fast, too high-pitched, too slow, or does it have normal rhythm and modulation? What are they not saying? We learn a lot the moment our patient says something – their region, and their educational, ethnic, and socioeconomic backgrounds often being immediately obvious. We obtain further clues about our patients' internal thought patterns by listening to their vocabulary, figures of speech, metaphors, and imagery, as well as looking for these three common language errors:

- A *deletion* occurs when some detail(s) essential to a complete understanding are missed out by the patient. For example, "I feel worse". Worse than what? In what way? Or "The whole lot are worried about Gramps". Who in particular? How worried are they? And about what in particular?
- A *distortion* occurs when actual behaviour and events are turned into protective abstract concepts which have no reality of their own. For example, "I'm suffering from my nerves". What does that mean? That you want more diazepam? That you want to see a psychiatrist? Or that the weekly trip to the supermarket is now a nightmare due to increasing agoraphobia?
- A *generalisation* means arguing from the particular to the general in a manner that excludes any possible exceptions to the rule they have made. For example, "I'm always getting headaches". Does that mean every week? Every month? Every day?

ACTIVE LISTENING

You will need to listen with genuine interest. This needs to be real and not fake. Work at it. Actively encourage the other person to talk by nodding, smiling, and echoing significant words. Show that you are listening and watching.

Reflect back in the patient's own words, not only to show that you understand, but that you are truly interested and hearing what they say. It also enables them to hear and understand their own meaning. But be wary of reformulating the patient's words. This can sometimes work well, but if you get it wrong the patient may feel alienated and be too afraid to correct you, leading to a mismatched agenda. It is important to do this in a highly sensitive and tentative way and seek clarification from the patient. Do not say something too abrupt which paints the patient as demanding or difficult: "So what you're telling me is you've had panic attacks for years and because they are not getting any better you want to see a psychiatrist?" Try "So let me see if I've understood you – your panic attacks have been a problem for a long time and you are wondering whether some specialist advice might help you cope with them better?"

Reflection can be a response to a cue. For example, the patient might say "and I've felt low this week", and the doctor might reply, "Low?" Equally, the same cue could be responded to by a later statement by the doctor: "You mentioned earlier that you felt low. Could you expand on that?"

Check what the patient has said. This can be done by giving them your interpretation of their story, inviting them to correct any misunderstanding and embellish the story further if needed.

Explain why you are asking a question. This can stimulate unexpected responses; for example, "The reason I asked about cramps and bloating was that I was wondering about irritable bowel syndrome" might be met with, "Oh, my sister's got that, and she said that's what I've got, but my mother reckons it's an ulcer".

Then, of course, there is the studied use of silence. This is often frightening to young doctors who, every time there is a pause, feel uncomfortable and duty-bound to say something, however inane. Try allowing pauses. The patient will invariably fill them if you wait long enough. Silence is something all doctors should cultivate. Not only does it actually mean we get more information, but patients perceive doctors who allow pauses for them to talk as being more understanding. Interactions with patients where the doctor actually says (and does) very little often rate as some of the most satisfying for patients. The ability to talk about their problems and concerns is frequently our patients' main reason for seeing you in whatever setting of medicine, though they often do not realise this themselves.

OBTAIN AND USE RELEVANT SOCIAL AND OCCUPATIONAL INFORMATION

You will need to establish the effect of the illness on the patient's work or home life. Clinicians often forget about such effects, but to our patients, these may be the main reason for them coming to see us. As continuity of care is decreasing, it is becoming even more important to find out this kind of information in every consultation. In those circumstances where you hope for some continuity of care, each time you obtain some personal information, you can regard this as a "brick", and over time you will build a wall. Make it a rule to know more about your patient when they leave than you did when they came in.

By now you should have a good idea of your patient's ideas, concerns, and expectations. You now want to form a working hypothesis and start to put some of your clinical pigeonholing skills into operation – what some might call the "proper" doctor bit.

b. Understand the Problem

OBTAIN ADDITIONAL INFORMATION ABOUT CRITICAL SYMPTOMS AND DETAILS OF THE MEDICAL HISTORY

First, you must obtain sufficient information to be sure that you are unlikely to miss any life-threatening conditions. Second, your verbal investigation should be consistent with your hypotheses, which you have now formed based on the information you have just obtained. This part is well taught in clinical training, and you will be well placed to focus in on the relevant aspects. You will naturally move into a more closed questioning style, and a patient having already been given the opportunity to explain what matters is more likely to respond succinctly, rather than needing to use your enquiries as opportunities to try to get across their agenda. It can help if you flag the change in style: "Thanks for explaining. I'm now going to ask some specific questions so I can get a better idea of what might be going on".

Even as you are testing your hypotheses, though, stay alert and actively listening. Valuable clues and cues can come at any point in the consultation.

ASSESS THE CONDITION OF THE PATIENT BY PHYSICAL INSPECTION IF APPROPRIATE

Any examination you choose should be one that is likely to confirm or refute your hypothesis or any other hypothesis that could reasonably have been formed on the basis of the evidence you have so far. Most good clinicians are aware that if they do not know the likely diagnosis after talking to the patient, the examination will rarely illuminate it – hence why a proportion of medical care can be undertaken remotely. However, most patients don't share this understanding; physical examination will be an unvoiced part of their expectations. There is an old adage: don't let a patient leave the consulting room without laying a hand on them. Even something as simple as taking a pulse or checking a blood pressure can have a powerful therapeutic (and theatrical) effect. In this era of remote consultations, if you don't think examination is necessary to reach a diagnosis and safe management plan, it is probably wise to explicitly explain this to your patient.

MAKE A WORKING DIAGNOSIS

Clinicians need to form clinically appropriate working diagnoses on which they can formulate further plans for investigations if necessary, or on which to base a management plan for their patient. In primary care, detailed clinical diagnoses are less common in the sense of the widely used disease model of medicine. The diagnosis becomes a flexible concept to allow the formulation of a rational and appropriate management plan. In hospital practice, where organic disease is more prevalent, the biomedical formulation dominates but beware the tendency for it to displace the psychosocial. The "hepatic failure in bed 6" is attached to a living, breathing human being with a life, a family, work, and interests, and hopes and fears for the future.

2. Share Understanding

Now think about the second half of the consultation. Getting the first half of the consultation right will give you the springboard to perform the second half well, but the tasks and skills involved are very different. Remember that this book is about learning to share in the consultation, *and the goal is to reach a shared understanding and a shared decision* with your patient.

Remember that explanation is a one-way process, from clinician to patient, whereas a sharing of understanding is a two-way process and it cannot occur unless personal details, health understanding, concerns, and expectations have been elicited in the first phase. Clinicians who are sharing understanding are also formulating management plans and strategies while they are talking and listening. The act of sharing understanding is intended to clarify, modify, and tailor the subsequent decisions, making them more appropriate to the individual. Much of the effective sharing will be in the emotional realm of wants, needs, fears, and irrational beliefs. Unemotional logic is not the stuff of most encounters. It is also important to realise that our patients' expectations of medicine's capacity to deliver diagnoses and cures will almost always outstrip the reality. This is a true understanding and one in which many patients will be reluctant to share.

Here we move to a higher level of skilfulness. Achieving a shared understanding does not mean always getting the patient to agree with you. It means that in order to achieve a genuine sharing you may have to agree with them. This may make you uneasy, and on occasions you may have to soften your views to try to keep a dialogue going. You cannot share with a monologue.

Share your Findings with the Patient

However involved they may be, the patient usually becomes passive and expectant while waiting for the revelatory pronouncements of the clinician. It is a skilful strategy to keep the patient involved: use their own words and continue to use the short-term memory of the previous exchanges. This explanation phase is the cornerstone of most consultations, and it often arises very quickly, even too quickly for many clinicians.

At this stage we should perhaps remind you that this is a book for clinicians. Good communication skills and bad medicine are dangerous bedfellows – do not forget the science that you have been taught. This book is about communicating that hard-learned science effectively, so by this stage of the consultation we hope you have got the medical content right. If so, now you must learn how to negotiate with the patient.

Tailor the Explanation to the Needs of the Patient

By now you know your patient a little. You should have a feel for the type of person they are, so that when you begin your explanation (and you should go first), you should ensure that your manner and language are appropriate to the patient's needs and that the information is presented in terms which they are likely to understand. You must tailor your explanation to the unique human being who is sitting in front of you.

Consider the following examples:

- "This rash is called psoriasis, and it is caused by overactive cells in the skin, but it is probably not affected by what you eat" (having elicited the patient's belief that the rash was due to an allergy to certain foods). "It usually comes from the genes, meaning it runs in families, which is why I was asking about your father's skin problems – I suspect he may have had the same. We do know psoriasis is aggravated by smoking, though".
- "You feel the new tablets are to blame for these symptoms. That is certainly possible, and if so, they should go away if we pause treatment for a couple of weeks. Shall we book a follow-up appointment for then? If you're better and still keen to try an antidepressant, we can look at an alternative, but I'd rather not start something else today – we want to be sure the symptoms settle; otherwise, we could end up confused. I know you weren't keen on psychological therapy before, but that could be just as helpful and without the risk of side effects – we can talk more about that next time, if you'd like".

Learn to speak the patient's language. Use short words and sentences as specifically as possible. Remember that the order in which information is given is important. Patients recall best what they are told first. Repeat important pieces of information.

A very common medical fault is to cloud explanations with technical medical jargon that is incomprehensible to almost everyone. Do not do it. The Academy of Medical Royal Colleges encourages doctors working in outpatients to write directly to patients and contains guidance on how to write such letters in order to improve patient understanding (Academy of Medical Royal Colleges, 2018). But a word of caution – avoiding jargon can make you sound very patronising, which is the reason it is a skill and must be carefully judged.

Learn to use appropriate delivery, which is how you say something, not what you say. It helps to use plural pronouns to indicate partnership. For example, "I hope you agree. Shall we meet again in two weeks to see how you are getting on?" Start by breaking information down into manageable chunks. Keep pausing and checking. Is the patient following what you are saying? Pace (the speed of delivery) is important. Try to match the patient's rate of speech. Eye contact is important. Keep watching for those cues. Try to match the patient's language of self-expression. For example, "You said you were 'absolutely knackered'. That's absolutely normal, an operation like you have just had is bound to make you feel that way".

Remember that understanding of words like "common", "possible", and "rare" can vary, and the use of percentages or other figures may be interpreted in very different ways. For example, patients are more likely to take a treatment such as a statin if they are told that it will reduce their risk of having a heart attack by a third than if they are told that it will reduce their actual risk from 12% to 8%. They will be even less accepting if they are told that the number of patients who would need to be treated for ten years in order to prevent one attack is 25. The important task is to convey such information in ways that are meaningful to the individual patient while not manipulating the message too disingenuously.

A good technique to learn and practice is "explicit categorisation". For example, "I am going to tell you what I think is wrong, what I expect to happen and which treatment I suggest". This may seem a bit military, but it is very effective.

Ensure that the Explanation is Understood and Accepted by the Patient

Clinicians quite enjoy giving explanations, but many appear to be given in order to make them feel that they have completed their own consulting process, and the patient is barely relevant. Ask yourself whether you are explaining for yourself or for your patient.

Again, remember to watch the patient's internal search. If you do not see the patient looking as if they accept what you say, continue to negotiate. The glassy-eyed, passive patient nodding obediently is not necessarily on board with the pearls of wisdom falling from your lips.

Watch for "non-verbal leakage". This may sound like a pool of muddy water forming around your patient, but it is actually the discrepancy between what your patient says and what their non-verbal behaviour is indicating. For example, "Yes, I will try the tablets", while breaking eye contact and squirming in the chair. You must act on these cues to be effective. For example, "You don't look convinced. Is there a different option you'd prefer?"

Actively encourage feedback, check your attitude again, and regularly check your patient's understanding, not least because it will probably increase your own. It is bad practice to give too much information, and don't get carried away by your own verbosity. A patient staring out of the window at the squirrels is a sure sign that you have gone on too long. Remember that much of what we tell patients they forget immediately, even if they understood or were listening in the first place. *They tend to remember what matters to them; this is often not what matters to you.*

Work from the MRCGP Consulting Skills module showed that checking patients' understanding was the rarest of all observed behaviours, with less than 5% of doctors demonstrating it. This means that it must be difficult to do. So how can you make it easier? Here are a few suggestions.

- It clearly implies the use of a question; for example, "Does that make sense?" But this is closed and invites a binary response, and "No" might feel too daunting.
- Better to try saying something like "I know today's discussion has been complicated. Would you tell me what you are going to tell your partner about what we have said?" or "We've covered a lot of ground. Would you like to tell me what you've understood?"
- If those approaches don't feel appropriate, giving opportunities for clarification can be just as useful: "Is there anything you'd like to ask me?" "Are there any things you're not sure about, or anything else you want to know?"

Some ask patients, "Can you explain what I have just said back to me?" We think this is too direct and a rather paternalistic approach that makes patients feel exposed. And the execrable "Is that an OK plan?" is just not good enough.

3. Share Decisions and Responsibility

Choose an Appropriate Form of Management

Your management plan needs to be appropriate to your working diagnosis. This is part of the knowledge and skills we are taught, and will be modified by your experiences throughout your career. Your management should of course reflect a good understanding of modern medical practice, and this is nowhere near as easy as it sounds. Medicine is ever-changing, the slavish demands of evidence-based medicine weigh heavily and litigation lurks in every corner. Uncertainty pervades all decisions. You can only do your best, and you must keep working at that.

Involve the Patient in the Management Plan to the Appropriate Extent

Patients should be involved in choosing their own management as much as possible, not least because their cooperation will be needed for the plan to be implemented. Management options should be shared with patients and, where appropriate, the patient should make the choice. This is another phase of explaining and sharing understanding, but this time it is about management, and the dialogue must be two-way. You may initially find this concept uncomfortable, but it is likely to make you more effective and less prone to "medicalise". Encouraging patients to see themselves as responsible for their own health may alter their locus of control a little and make them more likely to request information, as well as to use the medical profession more appropriately. Not all patients will want to be involved, and it is not always appropriate for them to be, but mostly it is. If your patient is involved, the risk of litigation and disagreement is much lower.

You may need to counter your patient's fallacious arguments and erroneous beliefs, and reinforce those beliefs that are helpful to the outcome. Try to foster patient autonomy and increase patient self-reliance. Remember that you are more powerful than you think you are, so use your power carefully. You must be prepared on occasion to admit to uncertainty, and this may not be easy for either you or your patient. Uncertainty is all-pervading – it is the worm in the apple of perfection. Your inner self is always in doubt, but this is the truth about being a clinician. Develop your humanity and learn to realise that uncertainty comes with the territory. Dealing with uncertainty is one of the hardest skills to learn in medicine; the earlier the phase of the illness, the greater the uncertainty. An experienced GP will cope with uncertainty much better than a newly qualified F1.

Sharing decisions need not be too onerous. For example, consider a patient with rotator cuff associated pain. You could say something like, "Well, you've had it a few weeks now. I think the best thing might be a cortisone injection – it's not too bad, you know. OK?" However, this is not sharing; it is telling. Alternatively, you could say, "Well, you've tried the gel but maybe a course of anti-inflammatories by mouth would be more effective. Physiotherapy can be very helpful, but it might take a while for you to be seen. Or what do you think about a steroid injection?" to which the reply might be "Er, well, doctor, what do you think would be best?" You might then say, "Well, it is not necessarily an 'either/or' – an injection could give you relief quite quickly, and when you get to see the physio you'd be better able to undertake exercise therapy". And so on. This is a dialogue.

Other examples of this approach include the following:

- "So, what do you feel about the strategies we have discussed?"
- "Would you rather start the tablets now, or wait a few weeks and see if it settles?"
- "I could refer you to a counsellor, or you could contact Relate yourself. Which would you prefer?"
- "Some people prefer to adjust their dose themselves. If I give you some guidance, would you?"

The extent of the sharing will depend on the patient, how capable they are of engaging in such involvement, the nature of the problem, and what types of options exist.

Consider the following examples:

- A retired science teacher with newly diagnosed hypertension might expect (or need) to be involved very substantially in a variety of options, ranging from lifestyle modification, through choice of drugs, to the frequency and nature of follow-up.
- With a patient with tension headache, you could discuss the treatments available, such as analgesics, relaxation techniques, referral for stress management, etc., and allow the patient to indicate their preferred course of action.

4. Make Effective Use of the Consultation

There are four pillars to ethical practice: beneficence, non-maleficence, equity, and autonomy. Shared decision-making is principally concerned with enhancing the last of these, but nothing we present here should be taken to downplay the importance of the other three. Patients may arrive with an established belief in the efficacy of a treatment you know has little chance of doing them any good, or they may have no sense of the potential for a drug or operation to cause them harm. They may believe that an expensive investigation like an MRI is essential to understand their longstanding mechanical back pain, but arranging it (were the radiology department even to agree) would in theory deprive someone else for whom that test would change management.

Most clinicians find conflict uncomfortable, and there is a natural tendency to shy away from conversations that have the potential to be contentious. But it is as fundamental a part of *shared* decision-making to introduce your professional judgements as it is to attend to your patient's perspectives. It may surprise you how often, once you have explained your views, patients will accept them and shift to meet you. You will have the greatest success in this regard where your exploration of their agenda has allowed you to develop a strong understanding of their ideas, concerns, and expectations, and where they have come from. And where there are no major concerns about beneficence, non-maleficence, or equity, your willingness to be flexible and support patient autonomy will be met with appreciation and a deepening of trust for future consultations. You will not always achieve the goal of a genuinely shared understanding and management plan, but where you have practised patient-centred medicine to the best of your ability, you can be confident that any such failure is ethically underpinned and represents sound medical practice.

Communication as a Competence: The Key to Avoiding Catastrophe

Countless enquiries and critical incident reviews have consistently demonstrated the fact that failures in communication account for more complaints and errors than any other single factor in medicine.

Of course, it is possible to be a good communicator, at least in the sense of being especially empathic and developing a superb rapport and therapeutic relationship, but still be a poor clinician. Communication is just one of the many skills required: it is almost impossible to be any good without it, but you can still be bad even if you do it well. Applied knowledge, pattern recognition, decision-making, and situational judgement are just a few other skills without which good communication remains just being nice to people. And patients can get that elsewhere.

Some of us wrongly assume that having got to this stage in our career we must be doing it right. Similarly, little external scrutiny is made of clinicians once they have completed their training, as they are presumed to have all the requisite competencies, including excellent communication skills. We typically get little or no feedback on our interactions with patients, either from our patients or from our colleagues, and consequently, we are rarely confronted by our shortcomings. Feedback on our performance is something we must actively seek, and for many, this is just too terrifying.

Evidence

Demonstrating effective communication with patients and relatives is a requirement in every medical training curriculum, and every doctor must now provide evidence of their ability to communicate effectively to revalidate. "Good communication skills" are seen by many as the Holy Grail of workplace-based assessments, which are increasingly the mechanism by which trainees are assessed. However, many give very little consideration to what their communication tasks actually are, what skills they need, or what they look like, and few really know how to recognise them in practice. It is very easy to produce "evidence" of communication skills and very difficult for anyone to prove that their abilities in this area are inadequate.

Assessing Communication

No one has yet clearly identified the magic ingredient that separates the novice from the expert in medicine. A good knowledge base and a willingness to listen and act on what the patient tells you is a start, but not enough. Experience can work both ways: if it shuts down the diagnostic search too quickly, it is unhelpful; if it allows exploration of paths not easily seen, it is useful. A simple guide to determine effective or less effective problem solving is to look at the time taken in the consultation to get to the point of examination when dealing with a new presentation. In most cases, the physical examination signals the end of the problem-solving phase, the examination is usually confirmatory, very seldom revelatory, and the explanation that follows is already decided. So, a very simple heuristic: the faster the examination occurs, the more fragile the problem solving. With complex problems, it is of course even more difficult; the most helpful skill in these cases is the ability to remain open to new ideas and information. The effective synthesis of all this information is what separates the diffident novice from the true expert, and the fact that some are better than others at this suggests that it is a subtle mix of the "science" of clinical reasoning and the "art" of good medical practice.

Most of us add to our factual knowledge cumulatively, and as we practise applying that knowledge a deeper understanding develops. As knowledge and problem-solving skills improve, problem-solving behaviours become more "expert-like". We do really have to emphasise the positive; yes, we make mistakes, but expert clinical reasoning is very likely to be right in the majority of cases.

When it comes to exams, communication is increasingly assessed through direct observation in standardised simulated situations. Assessment of communication competence relies on establishing what the measurable goals of the interaction are. Concepts such as "establishes rapport", "puts patient at ease", and "introduces self" are accepted, although rarely examined beyond the superficial. It seems for those who find this easy there is no need for examination, and for those who find it difficult there is little practical formative help available. Similarly, "demonstrates empathy" is a concept some find very difficult. Perhaps those who find this easy to demonstrate are particularly good at seeing things from the patient's perspective or maybe they are just better at acting?

Ways of Looking at Your Own Communication

This may be most relevant for medical students and those sitting postgraduate exams, but we believe that all clinicians could benefit from doing this, although we appreciate that many will not have the time or energy to do so.

The first problem with looking at your own communication with your patients is that you must *want* to do it, but nobody wants to look at their inept, stumbling, and wooden performances, do they? Why wear a hair shirt unless you are a monk? But you owe it to your patients and, what is more, if you learn to look properly you will find it fascinating, illuminating, and immensely rewarding.

What you want to achieve is a climate for true constructive formative feedback. Looking at yourself consulting is unnerving initially. Others looking at you can be terrifying. Why is this? There are several reasons. There is the fear of being found wanting, of being exposed, and of being attacked and ridiculed. So how can we create a protected environment? It is easy; there are just two rules.

Rules for Formative Feedback on Doctor–Patient Interactions

- Rule 1. Good points first.
- Rule 2. No criticism without recommendation.

There you are – simple! There is actually a third rule, which is *always obey the first two*.

Simple though these rules might be, that does not mean they are always easy to keep and enforce. Let us look at rule 1 first and imagine you are working in a little study group preparing for clinical exams. You have either role-played a scenario or are shown an actual recording of a consultation of yours. Your colleague starts the ball rolling with: "Great. OK, now what did you do well?" If you are not prepared for this question, you might easily demonstrate the "goldfish sign". A glazed look spreads over your physiognomy, your mouth begins to open and shut involuntarily but emits no sound, and your confusion has stymied your thinking. This is because you are not used to recognising what you did well. In all probability, you have been watching yourself with mounting self-disgust. But you did do well. You did many things very well indeed. You may need a little practice to recognise your strengths, but recognise them you must. Learning from watching yourself interact with patients must be a building exercise, not a destruction exercise.

If you are watching with a colleague or a teacher, you should start any discussion with what you did well. If you are having difficulty recognising your strengths, this is when your colleague or teacher can help. No criticisms should be made at all at this stage. Only when you have a thorough understanding of what you did well and the skills you used to achieve your strengths should you move on to areas where you think you were less effective.

We are very good at being critical. The problem is that our talent for supportive, formative, and constructive criticism is often underdeveloped. There is no place for criticism without recommendation. You may not agree with all of the comments, but you have been given some positive suggestions about your behaviour which you can use or not, and the discussion can be an open but sensitive one in which you are not unduly threatened.

Start using the rules now with your friends and try to persuade some of your teachers to follow suit. In our experience of groups, there is sometimes initial frustration at the constraints imposed by these rules, and someone will inevitably say: "Come on, Liz, stop pussyfooting about. Hit me with what you really think. What am I bad at?" The trouble with this approach is that eventually the teacher will relent and do just what has been requested. The result is obvious in the metaphorical sense. If you hit a human being hard enough they will always fall over, and that is what happens, and why the rules are there in the first place. Do not break them. Using such rules does not mean that you cannot touch on difficult personal areas and areas of special sensitivity. It just means that it takes time to create a supportive, trusting environment in which such delicate and meaningful discussions can genuinely take place to the considerable benefit of the learner, namely, you.

Real Patients

On balance, most patients do not mind being observed, discussed, or recorded, but there have to be rules and respect for the individual. Patients know when they go to hospitals that they will be seen more often than not by multiple clinicians. This is no excuse at all for the time-honoured medical practice of then discussing a fellow human being as if they were an antique clock, with the occasional excruciatingly patronising aside.

Patients are less passive in the less frightening and more familiar general practice setting and are more likely to assert themselves by refusing permission to be observed. If any form of recording (video, sound, or photo) of the consultation is to be made, obtaining watertight consent both before and after the consultation is vital, and this consent must be written. The EU's General Data Protection Regulation (GDPR) and the Data Protection Act 2018 have made the obtaining, processing, use, and storage of other people's (i.e. patients') data much more stringent. Your organisation will have a policy (or maybe several) on how to make recordings in compliance with the GDPR, along with the necessary consent forms. We suggest you follow this religiously, as any breach of the GDPR/Data Protection Act rules will be viewed rather dimly, and result in an inordinate amount of paperwork.

The most common method of recording is digital. Modern equipment is sensitive to low light, so will work in the dingiest of outpatient suites or surgeries. The on-camera microphones are good, but if you want better sound quality (and it is poor sound quality that ruins more recordings than anything else), you should use an external microphone. The aim must be to have both patient and clinician in shot with a clear view of their facial expressions. If you can only get one clearly, go for the patient.

Being Observed by a Colleague

Those working in hospitals do this all the time, but how many utilise this as a tool for improving communication? However, workplace-based assessments ensure that those in training must be observed talking to patients by senior colleagues at least sometimes. The feedback is supposed to be formative, although in many cases it is still treated as a test to be passed or failed, and little meaningful learning takes place. Emphasis in hospital inevitably falls on the content of the interaction (correct diagnosis and management) rather than the process. To improve your communication skills, you will have to find a like-minded colleague or trainer.

Simulated Patients

If you ever get the opportunity to work with actors or health professionals simulating real patients, do take it. You can obtain really useful feedback from an articulate, non-passive patient telling you what they really thought about your strengths and your less effective strategies. The wonderful thing about simulation as a learning tool is the fact that in real life it is almost impossible to know what any patient's "script" is. In simulation this is known, so you can see how far you got.

Simulation is also very useful for short-circuiting your learning circle, as it can produce particular patients with particular problems on demand.

Serious questions continue to be raised about the validity of the simulation assessment system, although the practical advantages compared to the old vivas and long cases are undeniable. We have some caveats, and what worries us is the encouragement of fast checklist behaviour to the exclusion of true curiosity about the human being in front of you. You cannot simulate curiosity – it simply becomes hollow acting and little else. So, learn how to consult to pass your exams, but please learn to consult properly as well.

Role-Play

Role-play is do-it-yourself simulation, and it can be very useful. Unfortunately, most people come out in a rash as soon as it is mentioned. It has always seemed to us that this fear is misplaced because, so long as the rules are strictly enforced, role-play has some safety valves built into it. The first of these is that it is artificial, and that is a legitimate defence for erratic performance, especially early on. The second is that we all vary in our ability to act, and being a terrible actor is not synonymous with poor medicine – the opposite also applies. The enormous strength of role-play is the occasion when you play the patient. Here you can really put yourself into their role and begin to understand what it feels like. This is worth much embarrassment and angst, and you really must seize every opportunity you get, as it truly will make you a better clinician.

A Last Thought, the Definition of Effective Medical Communication

This may be the biggest obstacle of all. Communication in medicine is not the ability to have a good chat; it must be related to diagnosis, treatment, and outcome. You will have to learn to share uncertainty and avoid pretending that you know everything. You will not always be popular. The task of most medical encounters is to achieve a reasonable shared understanding with the patient. Communication skills assessments are all very well, but they can easily just become shallow tricks of the trade without remembering their purpose. The purpose, as we have pointed out in this little book, is to tap into our patients' health beliefs while performing our medical diagnostic and treatment manoeuvres, and at the end of each interaction leave our patient as informed as their capacity will allow.

References

Academy of Medical Royal Colleges. *Please, write to me.* 2018. https://www.aomrc.org.uk/wp-content/uploads/2018/09/Please_write_to_me_Guidance_010918.pdf

Danczak, A. British GPs keep going for longer: is the 12 second interruption history? *BMJ* 2015;351:h6136. https://doi.org/10.1136/bmj.h6136

NHS England. *Improving communication between health care professionals and patients in the NHS in England Findings of a systematic evidence review and recommendations for an action plan.* 2021. https://www.england.nhs.uk/wp-content/uploads/2021/07/SQW-NHS-England-Improving-communications-report-30June.pdf

Index

I

K

L

M

N

O

P

For Product Safety Concerns and Information please contact our EU
representative GPSR@taylorandfrancis.com
Taylor & Francis Verlag GmbH, Kaufingerstraße 24, 80331 München, Germany

www.ingramcontent.com/pod-product-compliance
Lightning Source LLC
LaVergne TN
LVHW022108220926
848675LV00026B/259
* 9 7 8 1 0 4 1 1 0 9 6 6 2 *